No Match For Her

D1569347

TRAVIS LEE HICKS

No Match For Her

TRAVIS LEE HICKS

LilliSTRONG

Greensboro, NC

Copyright © 2019 Travis Lee Hicks
Front cover photograph by Travis Hicks
Back cover photograph by Fire Eye Studios
Dedication page photograph by Travis Lee Hicks
All other photographs by Travis Lee Hicks and Family
Book design and cover design by Travis Lee Hicks

All rights reserved. This book or parts thereof may not be
reproduced in any form, stored in any retrieval system, or
transmitted in any form by any means—electronic, mechanical,
photocopy, recording, or otherwise—without prior written
permission of the author, except as provided by United States of
America copyright law.

For permission requests or corrections, write to
travhicks@hotmail.com.

ISBN 978-1-7342517-0-8 (paperback)
ISBN 978-1-7342517-1-5 (eBook)
ISBN 978-1-7342517-2-2 (hardcover)
ISBN 978-1-7342517-3-9 (hardcover with dust jacket)

I dedicate this book to my family.
Y'all gave me the courage to write.

To **LouAnne**, I love you
unconditionally,
in sickness and in health.

To **Lilli**, **Amelia**, and **Collin**,
I am proud to be your Dad.
Your strength inspires me.
Y'all endured so much in youth
that you deserve the world as adults.

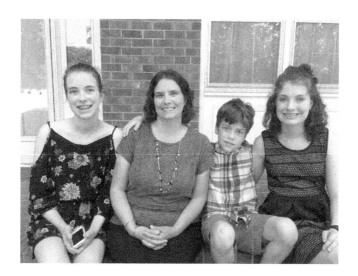

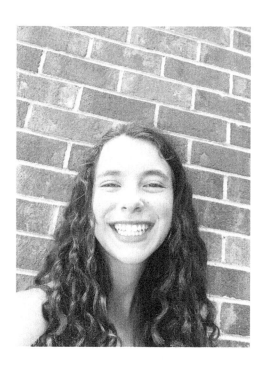

Foreword

By Amelia Hicks

Breathtaking. *No Match for Her* **is truly a breathtaking book. It** captures a journey of hope, bravery, courage, change, and inspiration. As someone who dreams of being an author, I was ecstatic to hear that my own Dad was writing a book. After a few months of his writing the first draft, I was the first one to read it. It was a Friday night, and once I sat down to read it I couldn't stop, reading it in one sitting. I cried, frowned, laughed, and smiled as I read this book. This book takes you on a journey of all emotions.

i

I was able to relive moments from a different point of view and with new light on things I went through. My Dad puts his life and soul in this book to share with others our family's journey. Whether you know my family's story or not, reading this book will allow you to picture events through my father's eyes. You will feel the emotions he felt. You will hear the things he heard. You will see the things he saw. This book will captivate you on this journey.

Knowing a loved one has cancer is life changing. Many people are battling cancer right now. Some won't make it, and others will have to worry about their cancers coming back for the rest of their lives. When I heard my Dad tell me, "Lilli has cancer," my life changed. I was terrified that my sister would die. I was scared of losing my best friend. I didn't want to believe it was true. This was the worst thing I have lived through; yet, it was also the most inspiring event. I was able to see life in a new light. I hope you all take this book and let it change your life for the better.

I am incredibly proud of my Dad. He had a dream of writing a book and made it real. This book is truly breathtaking and life changing. For all who read this I tell you that this is truly a masterpiece. Take this story to show you that life is a gift and should never be taken for granted. In fact, I challenge you to tell your loved ones how much they mean to you because you never know when it may be their last day. Thanks for reading this foreword, and I hope you all love this book as much as I do.

Introduction

....

Of all the books I've ever dreamed of writing – and there were many over the years – this is the last book I would've wished to have written. I never wanted to be the father of a cancer patient. Who would? After watching my daughter go through the fight of her life, I needed time to help my family regain some sense of normalcy. I couldn't bring myself to write much of anything.

I followed other pediatric cancer patients whom we knew from hospitals or from friends or friends of friends. After following a number of these kids—mostly on Facebook and other social media sites—and reading about how their stories continued beyond the hospital, I started writing down bits and pieces of my story as the father of a cancer survivor. I shared details of my experiences, along with updates about our daughter Lilli, via online posts during her various treatments. Following her treatments, I shared some of my reflections in a series of posts. From the positive feedback and encouragement that I got from friends and family and strangers, I decided to sit down and start writing this book.

When Lilli was first diagnosed with leukemia, I didn't want to hear many, if any, stories about folks who had such-and-such a cancer and how those people had dealt with their cancers. People were well-meaning, but I wanted to focus my energies on Lilli and her leukemia and not try to compare her to others who had fought their own battles against cancer. In time, I became more open to reading about other patients who were going through cancer treatments at the same time as Lilli. And much later I was finally able to read accounts written by people who had survived cancer or were parents of cancer survivors. I wouldn't say that I found comfort in reading these other accounts, as it was still difficult to follow stories of patients who might not survive (and some of them did not survive), but I could identify with the emotions of other parents of pediatric cancer patients.

I decided to start writing this work with the notion that there might be others out there who might read my words and either find comfort in or identify with my experiences as the father of a pediatric cancer patient. This book is for you, too, and for friends and family members of people facing life-threatening situations. I hope that you see in this book ways that you can support your loved ones while they go through their own struggles. It has not been easy to relive my experiences, but I have found some release from putting these experiences down on paper.

So here it is: my first book, a story about how my daughter's fight against leukemia was a wake-up call for me, a middle-aged man who was in the worst shape of my life when this story began. Years of sitting at a desk, mostly working on a computer as an architect and professor, and a lack of exercise left me overweight, out of shape, and lethargic. I had also become a workaholic, running on the tenure treadmill to generate a large enough body of work so as to deserve permanent tenure and a promotion from assistant to associate professor. I had lost sight of the important things in my life, like my health, family, faith, and time.

....

Before you begin this journey with me, I'd like to provide a few words of caution. First, do not treat this book as a healthcare manual. While I write about many medical procedures using lots of medical jargon in this book, I am not a doctor. I have written this work from my perspective as a layperson. You should see a medical specialist to address any health concerns you may have.

Second, do not follow any of the exercise routines that I mention in this book. I am not a certified trainer, dietitian, nor fitness guru, and I cannot guarantee anyone's health or safety as a result of attempting any of the routines that worked for me. If you are inspired by my story, then find a trained professional in your area who can help you in your own health and fitness journey, and consult your primary care physician before starting any exercise routine.

Part One

The Pillow Talks

I never would have dreamed it would be a pillow to break the news that my child had cancer, but that's how it happened. A pillow was the first thing, animate or otherwise, to deliver that blow…not a doctor or a nurse, and not in a consultation room or cancer clinic. It was in a dimly-lit children's hospital patient room in the dark wee hours of the morning where I found that pillow.

"Supporting families of childhood cancer patients," the pillow told me.

What a lovely pillow it was. It was a plush seafoam green pillow with a wishbone shape that would cradle a person's neck, made in a fleecy fabric, hand sewn with love, by volunteers (I pictured a quilting bee of little old ladies) from a church a stone's throw from Lilli's middle school. As if someone were reading Lilli's mind, there were silver dollar-sized owls inscribed in green circles. A hand-

1

made tag on that pillow delivered the devastating message that my Lilli-Bug had cancer.

Without letting Lilli see me remove the tag, inscribed also with the donating church's name and attached with a small safety pin, I put the evidence of her cancer in my pocket and tried to keep a straight and strong face. I couldn't let her see my true emotions, but I was scared.

I guess she really does have cancer. They probably won't tell me for certain, yet, because the doctor's not in.

If we were going to hear that news from the doctor, whoever he or she was, then I wasn't going to let Lilli see the same tag that broke the news to me. I would prefer she hear it from a doctor with experience talking to kids about these things.

Stay strong, Travis. Don't let her see you break down right now.

But I could tell that all the signs were there, including the tag on this pillow. The patient bed was adorned with this pillow, a Christmas-themed quilt, and a pillow case that all looked hand-made, not the kinds of things you'd expect in a run-of-the-mill hospital room where they only want to get you in and out of there as quickly as possible. Nope. There were also all kinds of life-saving valves, nozzles, gauges, monitors, and hoses mounted to the wall around the head of the bed, more than I had ever seen. And I had seen three different labor and delivery rooms over the years.

Yet there I was with my twelve-year-old daughter Lilli. I had just become a cancer parent, and she was a patient suffering from some kind of cancer that I would learn about later, once the doctor was in. We were both worn out from a sleepless night spent in the emergency department, having one test after another performed on Lilli before her being transferred to this patient room in the middle of the night. Even though we were worn out, Lilli couldn't find enough peace to fall asleep. She tossed and turned, coughed and wheezed, suffering from some kind of cancer. The nurses kept coming in and out of the room going through their checklists of things to do to get Lilli settled into her room.

I texted LouAnne to let her know the news, that it was some kind of cancer. Exactly what kind of cancer Lilli had was still unknown to us, and it would be hours later before we knew much more than what was on the pillow. Neither LouAnne nor I had slept, and we had been texting each other all night. We were both now cancer parents. The pillow told us as much.

Lillian Irene

....

Lilli is our first born. LouAnne and I chose the name Lillian after months of thinking about names, doing our research, buying and reading baby name books, and ultimately deciding on that name. We wanted to honor the memory of my mom Tracy (Honey) M. Hicks but struggled to figure out exactly how to do that. My sister Toni had already named a daughter Tracy Lynn after mom, and mom had legally changed her name from her given name of Threasa Marguerite to Tracy M. (no middle name, just a middle initial). Mom was strong-willed, and I interpreted her decision to change her name as an act of defiance. And anyway, my sisters and I called Mom "Honey" after we found that nickname in one of her old high school yearbooks when we went rummaging through her old wooden trunk. Honey made it hard for me and LouAnne to honor her with our baby's name.

We decided to honor Honey by using the name "Lily" after the flowers from which she made a living on a daylily farm in Putnam County, Georgia. In an effort to be different (Lily is one of the most common names now, but at the time it seemed fresh and different), LouAnne and I decided to use an older family name, Lillian, and abbreviate it to Lilli. We stuck with "L-I-L-L-I" despite LouAnne's misgivings about the spelling. With a name like hers, LouAnne knew what it would be like for future Lilli to continually correct people on the spelling of her name. Selecting a middle name proved easier for us, but we didn't completely decide on LouAnne's maternal grandmother's middle name, Irene, until we were in the labor and delivery room.

Lilli was born in Raleigh, NC, at the Raleigh Community Hospital. We were living in Louisburg—about an hour north of Raleigh—when Lilli came along. Without knowing anything about North Carolina, LouAnne and I had moved to Louisburg in 2000 to be close to Raleigh, a city we had researched and selected because of its career opportunities in architecture, music therapy, and teaching. "Louisburg? Lamar, that's where we're from," my great uncle Raymond had told my dad when he found out where we moved. Sure enough, LouAnne and I had been drawn to a fixer-upper in downtown Louisburg, a block away from where my ancestors had lived and a few miles from their final resting place. Chills went up my spine when I discovered that I was living that close to my kinfolk.

Life in Louisburg was romantic. LouAnne and I bought a 1915 two-story four-square house with a circular drive and porte cochère on a corner lot with huge oak trees. From this fixer-upper in the downtown historic district we walked to church, the

Louisburg Baptist Church, two blocks due east. Our next-door neighbor Miss Tommie, who turned 80 a week after we moved to town and still walked everywhere she went, was like our surrogate grandma. Other neighbors made us feel welcome, including my distant cousins we discovered after the local paper ran a story about our returning to my family's roots. Our phone rang off the hook after that front-page story.

Louisburg was small enough that its small-town hospital didn't deliver babies anymore. LouAnne found a great Raleigh practice of all women OBGYN doctors, and they looked after LouAnne closely because of her high blood pressure, which put her at risk for pre-eclampsia and potential difficulties during childbirth. We decided not to find out the baby's gender before LouAnne gave birth, so we had a boy's name picked out, too. Had she been a boy, Lilli would've been named Collin or Parker to honor the family names of our paternal grandmothers.

When LouAnne's due date approached, her mom, Janet, came up from Georgia to help us. She stayed for several weeks before and after Lilli's birth, and both she and LouAnne's dad, Joe, were there when LouAnne went into labor. LouAnne went into labor in the night, and the contractions continued for most of the following day. LouAnne and I had gone through the new parent training sessions offered by the hospital, and we had some ideas of what to expect. Nothing could've prepared me fully for the experience that was to come in Raleigh.

It was in the afternoon when LouAnne's contractions finally got close enough to each other that the hospital told us to come in. We brought our bags with all those things the instructors asked us to bring, and we even packed a portable CD player and some of our soothing Celtic music CDs. A music therapist by training, LouAnne made sure that music was part of the birth experience. We were assigned a small exam room until the contractions became closer still. Then, we moved into one of the larger full-service labor and delivery rooms. Dr. Gizzie was on duty at that time, and she remained calm and in control throughout the entire process.

LouAnne and I learned about the various medical devices that one could potentially experience during childbirth, but I didn't expect that we would get to experience nearly all of them during Lilli's birth. One of the devices, a long hat-pin-like tool, was used to assist in breaking LouAnne's water, which had not happened on its own. Another device, somewhat like a vacuum cleaner hose, was used to apply suction to the baby's head as it started to emerge. Yet another device was a giant set of forceps that Dr. Gizzie used to attempt to pull out the baby. The most important, yet scary, device to me was the heartbeat monitor that was attached to LouAnne's belly. It provided audible beeping that registered the baby's heartbeat, which was beating just fine until the contractions. With each contraction and push, the beeping from the monitor stopped momentarily. Beep. Beep. Beep...............Beep. While I'm no doctor, it didn't take much for me to figure out that the contractions were causing the baby's heart to stop, if even for just a second or two.

Shouldn't they be doing something about this? Is our baby going to die during this delivery?

7

The doctors and nurses showed some concern from the pauses in heartbeats, but they weren't as alarmed as I was. My heart practically skipped beats, too, as the monitor's pauses continued with each push and contraction.

LouAnne pushed for a while, and the baby's heartbeat stopped with each push. Dr. Gizzie looked at the nurses and then at LouAnne and said in a firm but caring voice, "We think that the baby is coming out at an angle and that the umbilical cord might be wedged against its head or body as it's trying to come out at this angle." The team proposed a change of course and an immediate C-section. After all that pushing and labor, now LouAnne would also have to go through the double whammy of a C-section.

The next steps happened at lightning speed and with precision in every movement. The team prepped LouAnne, handed me a kit with paper scrubs, hat, mask, and gloves, and walked us down the hall to the surgical suite. It didn't take too long from the time we walked into surgery until our baby was born. Standing beside where LouAnne lay, I looked over the sanitary blue curtain at the baby being held by the doctor, and I said, "It's a girl!"

"It's a girl," LouAnne beamed, as they gave me scissors to cut the umbilical cord and then handed our baby to LouAnne. She passed our girl back to the nurse, turned away from me, and vomited all over the floor. "That's pretty common. Don't worry about it," the nurse told me and then hurried me out of the surgical room after I kissed LouAnne's forehead. "I love you," I said, on my way out.

When I returned to the labor and delivery room, Joe and Janet were there to meet their first grandchild, a newborn baby girl pushed in by a nurse. While the delivery nurse performed the APGAR test—

another lesson learned from our prenatal classes—I paced the room, walking back and forth to the door to look outside the room and down the hall towards the surgery suite.

What's taking them so long? Now the baby is fine, but what about LouAnne? Is she going to make it through this?

The nurse opened up a huge closet that was hiding in plain sight the whole time. The wide doors opposite the bed opened up to reveal a small room that held more pieces of equipment and diagnostic devices for weighing, measuring, testing, and confirming that we indeed had a healthy, normal newborn. Aside from a stork's bite on her forehead, a v-shaped red mark where she had pressed against LouAnne's pelvis, and her being tongue-tied, the baby was perfect in every way. The nurse asked if I wanted to help give the baby a sponge bath, and I did, but I couldn't help but to worry about LouAnne.

After what felt like an eternity, the team wheeled LouAnne back to the room, describing how well she had done during the C-section and the surgery that came afterwards. She had lost a little more blood than some patients, and she required a higher-than-average number of stitches from the prolonged labor, but LouAnne was strong and healthy, too. I was a father, and LouAnne a mother. I didn't quite know what to do as a new Dad, despite having read all the parenting books I could find, but I was already in love with this most precious baby girl in the world. I spent the next day calling everyone in our address book, even distant acquaintances, to let them know that Lilli was born.

Two years later, almost to the day, LouAnne and I found ourselves back at the same hospital with the same doctor but a completely different kind of birth story. This time our daughter, Amelia Parker, wasn't waiting for anyone. She came in the middle of the night, not allowing time for LouAnne's scheduled C-section or even an epidural. She came on her own terms and at her own fast pace. And when Amelia was born, LouAnne looked over at me with tears in her eyes and said, "Happy birthday, Travis," as Amelia was born on my—I mean her—birthday. She's the best birthday present I've ever received. The nurses saw the tears, heard LouAnne, and said, "Aww, Dad, it's your birthday? What a special birthday."

When Amelia came along, we were in the process of moving from Louisburg to Cary, NC, to be closer to my jobs in Raleigh. I worked full-time as an architect and taught part-time in the architecture school at NC State in Raleigh. LouAnne had given up her full-time music therapy job after Lilli was born so she could work as a full-time stay-at-home Mom. The hour-long commute from Louisburg to Raleigh had become too much for me to justify. I was missing out on family time and needed to shorten my commute. We moved to Cary in 2004 with our two-year-old Lilli and newborn Amelia, and we found a new circle of friends and neighbors as we raised our girls in a new church and enrolled Lilli in the church's pre-school.

Three years and two weeks after Amelia's birth, LouAnne and I welcomed our son to the world at Rex Hospital in Raleigh. LouAnne's OBGYN team had changed hospitals, but we were all old friends by the time Collin Benjamin came around. His birth was totally different from his sisters. Because of the risk of pre-

10

eclampsia and low amniotic fluid levels, LouAnne's doctors planned to induce labor, which they did, and to coax Collin into this world. He came right on schedule, the result of perfectly-executed obstetrics, and he completed our family of five.

Lilli and Amelia grew up in the Greenwood Forest Children's Center, a preschool run out of our church in Cary. Lilli completed kindergarten and first grade at Fuller Elementary School in Raleigh before our family made another move in 2010, when we packed up for Greensboro, NC, an hour west. Following my dream of teaching full-time, I accepted a tenure-track assistant professor position at UNC Greensboro in the Department of Interior Architecture. We moved in the summer of 2010 with our young children and settled into Greensboro. We registered Lilli and Amelia at General Greene Elementary and Collin in the preschool at our new church, Guilford College UMC, and we began making new friends in our neighborhood, at church, and at schools.

Raking Leaves

The signs of pediatric cancer had been there for months if we had known what to look for. In October and November of 2014, our sixth grader, Lilli, had developed severe cold sores around her mouth. We took her to our pediatrician, Dr. O'Kelley, who prescribed some topical creams and suggested that cold sores are common enough but to keep an eye on them. Later the cold sores spread to Lilli's underarms. Dr. O'Kelley's advice was to keep applying the creams and for Lilli to be careful shaving her armpits. I had never seen anything like it, and I was mostly concerned about what other tween girls would think and say about Lilli's appearance.

What are the other kids at school thinking about her? She looks different enough to be made fun of. If she were in my class when I was in the sixth grade, I know a lot of students would've made fun of her. Middle schoolers can be cruel.

Lilli had just started sixth grade at Brown Summit Middle School, a magnet school for academic excellence. My own middle school experience was one of cliques, cruelty, bullying, taunting, and one big popularity contest. I couldn't bear to imagine what a mean-girls clique would do to someone who looked like Lilli with all those cold sores on her face. Lilli, on the other hand, didn't seem too phased by the cold sores except for wanting them to go away so she could feel better. And I didn't sense any bullying from her academically-focused classmates, thank God.

Lilli had also begun to lose energy that fall. I wasn't aware of the degree to which Lilli was losing steam, but I learned months later that Lilli had been falling asleep during school. The teachers might have thought this was par for the course for her, as it was her first semester at the school, but we would've been alarmed to hear that she was putting her head on her desk and falling asleep. Of our three children Lilli was the most energetic. She was the one who learned to stand and walk at the earliest age, and she was full of energy while awake. She would wake up in the morning and go full-steam until she lay down for sleep at night. This was not a girl who took naps in class.

One afternoon in November 2014, I was raking leaves in the front yard. We have two magnolia trees symmetrically flanking our yard. There are two huge red oak trees near the front corner of our house and even larger willow oak trees in our next-door neighbor's yard. Having magnolia trees means year-round raking, as they lose their leaves all the time and have annoying seed pods.

Why did we buy a house with two magnolia trees? TWO! I always hated picking up magnolia pods growing up with a huge magnolia tree in my front yard, and here I am the owner of a suburban lot with two of these beautiful—but frustrating—trees.

There were a lot of leaves to rake, and Lilli offered to help rake leaves after school that day. Lilli stepped out of the front door as the sun had already started to set and the porch lights were on. She joined me in raking, as she had done from time to time in the past, but she only lasted about five minutes before saying, "I'm tired, Daddy. I'm gonna go inside and rest." I thought maybe she was tired from middle school, from all the hard work she had to do to keep up with accelerated classes, but I didn't dwell on it. There were lots of leaves to rake.

The signs were there, but I didn't get it until we were in the hospital room the morning of December 13, 2014. 12/13/14 is a date I'll never forget. The pillow made sure of that.

A week before that pillow came into my life, I was preparing to play the pipes at church for the first time in a while, this time for a special Christmas service during the Advent season. The uilleann pipes, or Irish bagpipes, are one of my passions, and I can't turn down a chance to play them for others. The music director at our church had searched near and far and deep and wide to find a piece incorporating the Irish pipes, and she came across *The Winter's End*, a piece recorded by the great piper Liam O'Flynn, for me to play with some real musicians, hired guns whom our church would bring in from time to time for special events.

I showed up for a practice session at church with these real musicians, and I felt at home with this ensemble of guitar, cello, violin, pipes, and oboe, another double reed instrument like the pipes. None of them had ever played with an uilleann piper and were curious to know what this instrument was (a pretty common reaction to the Irish pipes), and the oboist commented that he felt his instrument was being reunited with a long-lost cousin in my pipes. We ran through the piece two or three times that Saturday morning, and I felt ready for the next day.

Our kids also practiced that Saturday morning. Lilli had a vocal solo from *Welcome to Our World* in the children's choir as part of the service, and Amelia was in that same choir. After I wrapped up my rehearsal I headed home while LouAnne practiced with the adult choir and heard the children's choir practice in the sanctuary. Later that day she said, "You should've heard Lilli's solo. She sounded so good."

"Oh, I'll hear it tomorrow morning in church," I said.

"Some of the folks in the adult choir told me she should audition for one of the local choirs in Greensboro. They told me she was an amazing singer," LouAnne added.

Sunday morning, I got up early, packed the pipes in the car, and headed to church. LouAnne and the kids came separately, as the pipes take up a lot of room in my car. I always pack an extra set of pipes (there's a bagpipe joke somewhere in that), my tin whistles just in case, a folding chair, and a music stand. I arrived early enough to tune up the pipes in the choir room before heading to the sanctuary, which was packed. Ushers had brought in folding chairs to fill the empty spaces and aisles for overflow. *The Winter's*

End was early in the service, so I headed to the pulpit area with the other musicians, tuning and getting ready for the service to begin. The kids had gone to rehearse in one of the classrooms while I was warming up with the ensemble.

Just before the service began, LouAnne came from the choir room down to the edge of the pulpit. "Lilli got sick in the bathroom, and she's not gonna do her solo," she said. I got no more details than that.

I'm sure she doesn't have stage fright! She's used to singing in public and to having solos, but I wonder what happened.

"It's not like my daughter to get stage fright," I told the guitarist I had met the previous day, and then I noticed that Lilli had come in to the sanctuary with one of the minister's families sitting behind the last pew in a folding chair. She didn't look well, and she appeared crushed that she wasn't going to be able to sing her solo.

The Winter's End went off without a hitch, and I was relieved that my pipes sounded as good as they did on a cold dry morning. As soon as we finished, I walked from the pulpit and headed back to sit next to Lilli. I didn't know what was going on inside her body nor what happened in the restroom, but the seating was so tight that morning that I had to put my arm around her for the remainder of the service. I felt unusually close to her that morning. The children's choir did a great job as usual. Lilli didn't sing her solo, but one of her friends came through and sang a beautiful solo in Lilli's place. After the service, LouAnne confirmed that Lilli had thrown up in the church's restroom. "We should probably let them know to clean up the bathroom stall," LouAnne said.

16

Lilli started running a fever later that day, and she had not shaken it by the following morning. She stayed home from school, and LouAnne took her to the pediatrician's office. It was early December, the time of year when folks come down with colds, other viruses, or the flu, and the pediatrician couldn't quite figure out what was going on. Dr. O'Kelley suggested that we give it a few days and come back if things did not improve. Lilli stayed at home in bed that day, and I figured that it was some kind of bug she caught at school.

Lilli lay in bed for several days and nights, fighting this fever, a more lethargic version of our LilliBug than I had ever seen. On Wednesday, after two more days of a fever that wouldn't break, Lilli and I headed to Dr. O'Kelley's office for a follow-up. He took another look at Lilli and tested her for more things like the flu and strep throat. Still negative. He was stumped but prescribed an antibiotic to help with whatever was causing the fevers. He also asked us to come back Friday for some additional tests, including a blood test, if Lilli had not improved by then.

When LouAnne got home from work she asked about the doctor's visit and how things were going. Lilli's fever still was not subsiding, and all the tests had come back negative. LouAnne had done lots of research online, searching for information about all kinds of illnesses. I had not thought about cancer up to that point, but LouAnne said, "I'm worried. If she keeps having this fever and nothing helps, then it might be leukemia from what I've read online." That was the first time either of us uttered the word *leukemia*.

"Ssssssshhhhh! It's not that, LouAnne," I said. "Stay positive. It'll get better." In the back of my mind, however, I thought that she might be right and that there could be something seriously wrong with Lilli.

What if she's right? What if Lilli really does have something as serious as leukemia? And what do I know about leukemia? I don't know anyone who's had leukemia, at least not that I recall. Don't think about that, Travis. There's no way she's got leukemia. She's our kid who never gets sick.

For several more nights, Lilli struggled to sleep. She was up most of each night tossing and turning, coughing a deep and heavy cough most of the night. To this day, I hear those coughs in times of stress and anxiety. I lay in bed at night listening to her coughing from her and Amelia's shared bedroom at the other end of the hallway. The fever remained, off and on, and Lilli was warm to the touch except when she managed to sweat out the fever a few times.

On Thursday, I hosted a pot luck at UNC Greensboro. Lilli's health was on my mind as I had shared her updates with students. One of my students, a former nurse, and I talked about Lilli. Without knowing how serious it was, the student and I talked about dietary changes that could improve Lilli's overall health. I was frustrated that Lilli wasn't getting better, and my student didn't have any better ideas than the pediatrician.

By Friday, Lilli was no better, but I had a prior commitment that morning, leaving LouAnne to take care of Lilli. I drove over an hour to Mocksville, NC, to play Christmas tunes on the pipes, whistles, and concertina for the seniors' group at Blaise Baptist

Church. One of the members there heard me play earlier that year at the Davie County Senior Center and scheduled me to play months in advance. After finding the senior group having breakfast in their fellowship hall, I sat and chatted with a few of the churchgoers while sipping coffee and thinking through my tunes. Then, we headed over to the modest church sanctuary where I played for an hour, going through a selection of religious and Christmas tunes. In spite of a solid performance, I was thinking about Lilli the whole time. LouAnne texted me updates all morning about what was going on.

LouAnne took Lilli that morning to see Dr. O'Kelley, but he was out. Instead, they saw a different pediatrician who was about to send Lilli home like the other times that week. LouAnne persisted and demanded a blood test as Dr. O'Kelley had recommended. She called me to tell me that she was taking Lilli to a lab near the women's hospital and asked me to stay with Amelia and Collin. When LouAnne came home that afternoon she said that the labs were ordered "STAT" and that the doctor's office would give us a call if there was anything to be concerned about. I was worried about the potential results, but my confidence in Lilli's health increased with every passing minute without a phone call.

After dinner, I settled into the recliner in the den in the basement, with the TV on in the background, and sat down to grade some papers from school.

If they found anything in her labs, then certainly they would've called us by now. I think we're in the clear. They would've called by now, right?

19

After working for about an hour, I could hear LouAnne upstairs talking on the phone in a very serious tone. I heard the concern in her voice as she walked down the stairs and said, "I can't talk right now. I'm handing the phone to my husband." By that time, it was about 9:30 on a Friday night. The doctor on-call from our kids' pediatrician's office said, "Mr. Hicks, I was informing your wife that we'd like you to take Lilli to Brenner Children's Hospital as soon as possible. We would like to rule out things like leukemia. The labs came back, and Lilli's extremely high white blood count indicates something is off."

I realized my role was to be strong, firm, and steady while my world was moving and spinning in slow motion as I processed what the doctor was saying. If Lilli really did have leukemia, then we had to get her the help she needed, as the doctor ordered.

"What's the name of the hospital?" I asked, "And where is it? How do I get there? And where do I go when I get there?"

The doctor on the other end was calm, but he sensed the severity of the news he had just delivered. In a soothing voice, he gave me directions to the hospital, the exit number to take, and a general description of the emergency department of the children's hospital. He told me to pack a bag for Lilli, and that she would most likely be there a few days for some additional tests.

"You'll have to drive her," LouAnne said. She was a nervous wreck by that point and didn't want to be the one to drive the half hour to the hospital that late at night. We walked upstairs to deliver the news to Lilli while she, Amelia, and Collin were getting settled into bed.

"Lilli, the doctor's office called," I said. "They want you to go to the hospital, and you'll be there a few days for some tests."

Lilli and I took showers, not knowing when we'd be able to shower again. Lilli showered first, and LouAnne and Lilli packed a bag while I jumped in the shower. I emerged from the shower, looked in the mirror, and shook uncontrollably. I had to be strong in front of Lilli, but in front of this reflection I gave myself permission to be emotional for just a moment.

Leukemia? Did he really just say "rule out leukemia?" LouAnne might've been right a few days earlier when she suspected something was seriously wrong with Lilli. God, please don't let this be leukemia!

I dried off and got dressed, pulled myself together, and made sure that Lilli was ready for the trip. She packed a grey roller bag with a change of clothes, some toiletries, a book she was reading for school, and a purple stuffed owl named Violet. LouAnne and I held each other tightly before I took off with Lilli, and we agreed to keep texting each other updates. My body felt twice as heavy as usual, as each movement became more difficult and labored. It took all I could muster to go through all the motions of packing, walking, talking, and driving.

Wearing our warmest clothes and heavy winter coats, Lilli and I jumped into my Mazda 5 to drive the half hour to Winston-Salem around 11:00pm on Friday, December 12, 2014. I was numb to the temperature, and I was numb to the drive to Winston. Lilli sat in the front seat beside me, using my phone to navigate along the way, but she was weak and sick, holding onto her stuffed owl and trying to rest despite coughing.

I prayed silently during the drive that there was some kind of mistake in the labs and that we would get better news than that Lilli had leukemia. As I looked over at Lilli and how lethargic she was, I feared the worst.

What if this is the last time she ever sees the outside world?

Emergency Room

....

Cloverdale, Exit 4. That's the exit the doctor mentioned. We approached it, and I could sense the magnitude of the place before we ever made it to the parking deck. Sitting flush with the Interstate 40 business route, the hospital was an expansive collection of architectural additions, glowing in the crisp winter air. There were colorful lights and curvy lines that we could see from the car and a clear storefront entrance to the emergency room lobby with glowing red letters that declared, "Brenner Children's EMERGENCY." At such a late hour finding a parking space was no problem, but we newcomers took a while to navigate the maze of interconnected parking decks to find a spot close to the emergency room. I felt small as we exited the parking deck, walked the cavernous space between tall towers and parking structures, and headed towards the emergency department entry tucked under a pedestrian bridge.

Checking into the emergency department around 11:30, I submitted my insurance card, informed the receptionist of the doctor's sense of urgency in our getting there and of Lilli's elevated white blood count, and found a place to sit and wait. Lilli and I were not alone in the waiting area, but we found breathing room in a corner, where I took a selfie of the two of us and texted it to LouAnne to let her know we made it. Lilli managed a half smile while looking pale, weak, and frail.

Soon the staff called us back to an exam room, where the nurses took Lilli's vitals and started an IV for lab draws and to push fluids. The room was efficient but small, just large enough for a bed, a guest chair, a stool for the doctors and nurses, and a small wall of cabinets and sink. A TV mounted high in a corner of the room would entertain us for a few hours, although I was too stressed to pay much attention to it. Our common denominator that night was the Food Network, which had an all-night marathon of *Diners, Drive-Ins, and Dives* with Guy Fieri. It would take several years after that night before I'd voluntarily watch another episode of *Triple D*, as I associated it with the worst night of my life.

There we were: a twelve-year-old girl, her forty-one-year-old father, a stuffed owl, a school book, and a rolling suitcase in a small emergency department exam room. Lilli commented on how sterile it was, how whoever designed it clearly didn't understand children. "This is such a boring room, Daddy. They really should redecorate," she said. As an architect and interior designer, I couldn't agree with her more. Except for one wall painted green and a few token colorful floor tiles, the room was sterile, dull, lifeless, and one of the last places you'd want to be with a sick kid in need of healing.

We were stuck there for four or five hours while the staff performed various tests on Lilli, mostly drawn from her IV. At one point, they asked for a urine sample. Attached to an IV pole, Lilli needed some help to get to a restroom where she could provide this sample. I felt awkward as the Dad who had to take his tween daughter to the restroom and help her with all the tubes and such. When our girls had gotten old enough to bathe themselves, I stepped back from my fatherly duties of helping them bathe and get dressed. But here I was in a small emergency room washroom helping Lilli collect a urine sample.

Keep your cool. You can do this. You have to remain strong for Lilli's sake.

Helping her collect urine in a plastic bottle would be a cake walk compared to things in store for me and Lilli further down the road.

Lilli also had a series of X-rays, which required a wheelchair ride down a different hall to the radiology suite, and a number of blood tests. At one point a kind young nurse came in and let me know that they had tested for mononucleosis (I was hoping and praying that it would be something like mono), but that it was looking more serious. She then caught herself mid-sentence and said, "Oh, they haven't told you a diagnosis yet?"

I don't think anyone in here is going to tell me what's going on with my daughter. I guess they're trained not to give results, like x-ray technicians who really "see" but can't "say" what's on the x-ray. Lilli's calm about it, so I'll stay calm, too.

Lilli and I made small talk about school, about her assignments and about what she had missed the previous week while she was out sick. Lilli was concerned about missing school and talked about how she couldn't wait to get back. It was Saturday morning by that point, and Lilli had calculated when she might return to school if the pediatrician's office was correct in suggesting that we'd be in the hospital for a few days of tests.

"Maybe I'll be back by Tuesday," Lilli said, "or Thursday, or Friday at the latest. They mentioned that I might be here a few days."

I knew that Tuesday would be out of the question. By that point I had already Googled "childhood leukemia" and had some idea of what we were in for if our worst fears were realized. I couldn't let Lilli know that I had researched this and found that the treatment plans for pediatric leukemia would be extensive and risky.

I couldn't bring myself to open up to Lilli, but I had been texting LouAnne all night with updates about the various tests. I could open up to her.

"I'm scared," LouAnne texted.

"I'm scared, too," I replied, "I love you."

We didn't yet know what was going on inside Lilli's body, but the staff kept talking about admitting Lilli to one of the upstairs rooms so that she could undergo additional tests over the following few days. They kept referring to the doctor on call that weekend and suggested that she would be in later Saturday morning when we would learn more about Lilli's diagnosis.

It was about 4:00 or 5:00 in the morning when we finally escaped the exam room. "We're going to transfer you to a patient bed upstairs," a nurse said. She unlocked the wheels on the bed, attached the IV fluids to an extension pole on the corner of the bed (I hadn't noticed that pole until that moment), and started wheeling Lilli through the emergency department to a maze of corridors that seemed like the back-of-house circulation for hospital staff. All the corridors were dark, dull, and empty at that time of day, and it was a lonely walk from the emergency room to the elevator. I pulled the suitcase behind us and went with Lilli and the nurse to a large staff elevator, bright as the sun in comparison to the hallways, and up to yet another maze of dim corridors that led to a unit with a nurses' station and private patient rooms. The nurse badged in to a card reader beside a pair of locked doors, and the doors' motors whirred, opening the doors in our direction. After going through those doors, we were inside a locked unit, on some upper floor of the hospital.

We were, as it turned out, on the 9th floor in a pediatric hematology-oncology unit of Brenner Children's Hospital (part of the larger Wake Forest University Baptist Hospital complex), with sixteen patient rooms. It was in one of those rooms that a pillow gave me a definite answer to the question, "Does my daughter have cancer?" which the emergency department staff seemed instructed not to do. I looked around the room to find a clinical-looking sofa that doubled as a bed for visitors, a wall full of life-saving devices, a larger patient bed, a built-in closet and cabinet with a TV, and an adjoining bathroom. A nurse offered me a pillow and blanket, which I took, and I laid on the vinyl sofa pad to try to rest. Lilli was transferred to the patient bed with the donated pillow, Christmas-themed quilt, and special pillow case.

As I dozed in and out of sleep, I was awakened by nurses and aides who constantly came in to check on Lilli, to draw more labs, and to administer IV meds and fluids. With each visit from the staff Lilli would call out to me, "Daddy!" a cry that will stay with me the rest of my life. She was scared by all the pokes and jabs and from being a small patient in a big room. I tried to reassure her that the nurses were there to help her feel better, and I trusted them to do their best. I was exhausted, and I knew that I needed to rest so that I could be awake later when LouAnne and others showed up.

Dinner Guest

I had heard over the years that in times like these people get angry at God, ask God "Why me!?" or even turn their backs on God. I had been in enough Bible studies over the years, particularly the ones I took with Mickey Efird through the Duke Divinity School's Lay Academy, to understand that God was not the cause of my pain. I didn't believe that God had caused Lilli's cancer. I didn't believe that "everything happens for a reason," either, even though I would hear that expression a lot over the following few years. I did believe that cancer was real, that cancer happened both randomly—in the case of leukemia, as a result of bad habits like smoking or dipping (I was from the South, after all), and by environmental causes like asbestos. Bad things like cancer could happen to good or bad people, and who was to say whether I deserved the "good" label or the "bad" label? Or both?

I thought back on a time in the late 1990s when LouAnne and I lived in Lawrenceville, New Jersey, before we thought about having children. I had been out of graduate school a few years, and LouAnne and I both had good jobs in the area. We lived between Trenton and Princeton, in an apartment behind and above a cobbler shop run by Frank Cervone, whose family had built the building and who had grown up in the apartment himself. In the summer of 1998, we invited a missionary for dinner so that we could learn more about what she was going to do in the mission field. We got acquainted over dinner, after which she said, "You really have lived a perfect life." I didn't know how to react, as I didn't know her well enough to read her, and I went with the flow and responded, "I guess we have been blessed."

A perfect life? How can a perfect stranger presume to know so much about us from one dinner conversation? It's been a good life, but not perfect by any means.

LouAnne and I were a match made in a flower bed. We met when we were in elementary school, growing up in neighboring counties in middle Georgia, because our parents had a shared interest in flowers, mainly daylilies and irises. In high school, I took a romantic interest in LouAnne. How could I resist her blue eyes, wavy brown hair, and sweet personality? We were high school sweethearts and started dating around the time of junior prom. I called her younger brother Danny before the prom and asked if he thought LouAnne liked me and if he thought she might go to the prom with me. Before I could stop him, Danny put down the phone and said, "LouAnne! Would you go to the prom with Travis?" WAIT, I wanted to say, but when she said yes, I thought, "that didn't go exactly as planned, but...she said YES!" You could've knocked me over with a feather for weeks after that. LouAnne and I dated for the rest of high school, and I was convinced that she was the girl for me when she was hospitalized in high school with a bad case of mono. I visited her in the hospital, saw her frailty, and couldn't imagine my life without her. I knew at that point that I'd one day ask her to marry me.

I worked very hard in high school, discovered my love for architecture—or at least what I thought was architecture—in Mr. Stokes' drafting class, and was awarded a full scholarship and several additional scholarships to study architecture at Georgia Tech. I worked hard at Tech, and my hard work paid off when I was accepted by the School of Architecture at Princeton on a full fellowship. LouAnne lived at home while working hard at her hometown school, Georgia College, where she studied music therapy. LouAnne and I got married between our junior and senior years of college, and I studied abroad in Paris during my senior year. LouAnne spent some time in Paris with me, and we moved to Princeton once I was back in the States. After graduation, we were both successful in finding jobs in our areas of expertise straight away.

To this missionary dinner guest our lives must've sounded perfect, but I also heard in her comments a bit of jealousy or envy. Over the years, her comments and tone have stuck with me, carrying more weight in my memory than I should allow them, because my life has never been perfect. I've had my share of ups and downs over the years, and why would anyone expect to know everything about someone else's life from one meal? Perhaps I should've let this dinner guest know that I never got to know any of my grandparents very well, that my father's brother died when I was a young boy and that his death haunted me for years, or that I had to work extremely hard and make personal sacrifices for all those academic successes. I didn't say any of those things that evening, but I've made a conscious effort over the years not to jump to conclusions or to make assumptions about how easy or hard someone's life has been.

Within a year of that dinner guest's comments I experienced what, to that point, was the worst day of my life. It was my and LouAnne's five-year wedding anniversary. We decided to take the day off work and to go somewhere different. We went to Longwood Gardens near Philadelphia, a short drive from our apartment, and we spent the day checking out the flowers and landscape design of the garden and having lunch on the grounds. Our parents' passions for flowers must've worn off on us.

When we got home we walked upstairs to our small corner living room. The little red light was flashing on our answering machine. The first message said, "Travis, this is your dad. Your mom was taken to the emergency room in an ambulance. Give me a call." What?! This was in the days before any of my family had cell phones, so I had to find someone back home who was near a land line. We called the hospital and were able to connect to my dad who sounded very concerned. "Your mom's in bad shape, son. You need to come home." Dad told me that Mom had been found unconscious by my brother-in-law, Wayne, and that she had been taken initially to the local hospital before being transferred by ambulance to Piedmont Hospital in Atlanta.

It was already late in the afternoon when LouAnne and I learned all this and decided to drive to the Philadelphia airport and hop on a plane to Atlanta. Our flight was delayed, and we arrived in Atlanta late at night. LouAnne's mom and brother, Danny (the matchmaker), picked us up from the airport and drove us to the hospital. Once there, we went to Honey's room, walked in, and found an empty bed, neatly made up as if no one had laid in it that night. In this patient room my dad, sisters, brothers-in-law, an aunt, and an uncle were all there with puffy red eyes.

I knew instantly that Honey had not survived whatever caused her death earlier that night. I hugged Dad and sobbed uncontrollably. I awoke that morning with an anniversary celebration on my mind, and I went to bed that night in my old house in Georgia with one fewer parent. I had to be there for Dad and my sisters while we worked through questions like, "What kind of casket would you like?" and "Who'll be pall bearers?" Mom's life's work, a farm full of daylilies, was in full bloom and at its most beautiful on the day of her funeral, and the church was packed with folks of all different backgrounds, reflecting Mom's acceptance of all different kinds of people. Her older brother, Bobby, from Arkansas, who hadn't visited us in years, said, "I'll have to go home and do some soul searching. If she was able to do all this with her life, then what'll I do with what I've got left?"

That was the worst day of my life up to that point. A perfect life was far from my reality. My mother would not live to see any of my children. Knowing that one of her grandkids would have cancer at the age of twelve would have been devastating to her.

After Honey passed away I poured almost all my spare energy into new musical instruments. I had become smitten with the uilleann pipes during a Chieftains concert in March of 1999, a few months before Mom passed away. The concert began with an uilleann pipes slow air solo played by Paddy Moloney, leader of the Chieftains. I leaned over and whispered to LouAnne, "I'm going to do that," without even knowing what "that" was. Once I figured out what his mesmerizing instrument was called and learned that a piper was living no more than 15 minutes from our apartment, I was set. Fiddle player and piper, Fiona Doherty, moved back to Ireland following my second lesson with her, and I connected with Willie and Siobhan Kelly of Boonton, New Jersey. Siobhan taught me the tin whistle and Willie the pipes in what was the most productive year, musically speaking, in my life.

I now play three different sets of pipes made by some of the best pipe makers on the planet, like Benedict Koehler and David Quinn, but as a father and a husband I have less time to play music than I did when I first strapped on a set of pipes in a pipe maker's workshop 20 years ago. I play in church and for community groups who find out by word-of-mouth about my unusual instruments. I still play tin whistles in all different keys, and I occasionally play the anglo concertina, having owned, bought, and sold antique and modern concertinas over the years.

It's hard to say if I have a "worst day" of my life anymore. How would one decide what's worse: not being able to say goodbye to a dying mother or finding out your daughter has cancer? They're both "really" horrible, awful things for anyone to endure, and I wouldn't wish either of them on my worst enemies.

Diagnosis

Around the break of day on December 13, 2014, I met the pediatric oncologist who was on call that weekend, Dr. Marcia Wofford. She was a kind and compassionate doctor who spoke with authority and tenderness. She sat down in the chair beside Lilli's bed, between me and Lilli, and told us that Lilli was a very sick girl with leukemia. Dr. Wofford said that she had not yet looked at the blood samples closely enough to tell exactly what kind of leukemia it was but that she would be studying them later that morning. She said that Lilli could look at pictures of those cells if she wanted, and Lilli said, "no," that she wasn't interested. She was more concerned about missing school.

Lilli was calm considering that she had just found out that she had cancer. I tried to play off Lilli's emotions and remain strong for my daughter. We asked about the different kinds of leukemia that Lilli could have, and Dr. Wofford educated us on the two main kinds of leukemia. She told us that most of her pediatric leukemia patients had Acute Lymphocytic Leukemia (ALL), a kind of leukemia that would require three years of chemo treatment, mostly through outpatient treatments in the oncology clinic, including maintenance chemo. She said that about 20-25% of her leukemia patients had Acute Myeloid Leukemia (AML), which would require a more intense, but shorter, chemo regimen of 4-5 months. She explained that doctors didn't know what caused leukemia but that they had come a long way in treating this cancer during her years of practice.

After Dr. Wofford left the room, Lilli and I had some time to let these treatments play out in our minds. If ALL, then Lilli would go through treatments for all three years of middle school and would then be finished with treatments by the time she got to high school. If AML, then Lilli would have chemo for the rest of sixth grade but would then be finished with treatments in time to go back to school by the time seventh grade would start in the fall. Lilli's preference at that time was to have a shorter and more intense treatment because it would allow her to get back to school. I feared that a more intense chemo regimen must have some justification that I didn't want to hear.

LouAnne and I had texted each other throughout the night, and she was making plans to get help from friends and neighbors with Amelia and Collin so that she could come to the hospital. Our friends and family were waking up to the news about Lilli. We had shared our ordeal with our Sunday school class from church through our private Facebook group. Word had gotten out in the church, and Lilli's youth minister had contacted the senior pastor from our church, who knocked on Lilli's door that morning.

I went to the door to find the senior pastor on the other side. He had been a hospital chaplain at one time, and he was very familiar with the hospital and the surrounding area. I told him that Lilli had leukemia and that we still didn't know what kind of leukemia it was. "Leukemia…now THAT'S a scary word," he said. I couldn't say much in response, as I was still in shock and couldn't begin to form words into sentences without choking up. He could sense my emotions' getting the better of me and proceeded to pray for Lilli and our family, offering to help by getting the word out in the church.

Shortly after the pastor's visit there was a flurry of activity in Lilli's room. The nurses came in and said that they were moving Lilli to a different room down the hall, a pressurized room that was more isolated and separated by an airlock with a sink for washing up before and after visits. I should've been suspicious of this transfer, but I didn't think much about it at the time. All of this was a shock to me, and the subtleties of healthcare and the distinctions between different tests and procedures would be lost on me for a month, at least.

The first room had a great view of a wooded neighborhood near the hospital. There were several neighborhood churches with steeples that emerged from the treetops, and I could feel a connection to God and to others by looking out the large picture window that stretched wall-to-wall. This second room was larger and had an airlock that provided a bit more privacy from the shared corridor on the unit, but the view was much different. The room was on a different side of the building and had a view of a commercial strip with a Harris Teeter super market, the parking deck where I had parked the night before, and the busy highway from which Lilli and I had taken the Cloverdale exit. I had to search the landscape for signs of God and community, and I found them off in the distance in a distant steeple and a few house rooftops, barely visible.

The staff changed their appearance upon our change of rooms. In the first room, the nurses came in and out in their scrubs, but as soon as Lilli was transferred to the second room, they came in dressed out in hazmat-looking suits of paper, plastic, and rubber that covered their heads, bodies, shoes, hands, and faces.

WHAT?! What is it about Lilli that has these folks dressing like she has the plague?

After months of spending time in the hospital I would learn that these outfits were precautionary and were there for the good of the other patients on the unit who were susceptible to catching random viruses, bacteria, and fungal infections from one another, but I was freaked out by watching people take care of my girl as though she had ebola. Through all of this, however, I had to maintain my strength and stability in front of Lilli. She was a solid rock of little to no emotion, and I tried to follow suit.

LouAnne arrived shortly after they transferred Lilli to the pressurized room. Like me, LouAnne had to remain calm and strong for Lilli, trying not to break down in front of our oldest of three kids. LouAnne hadn't seen Lilli in a hospital bed like this, and she had to sit on the edge of the bed and hug her baby girl for a long time. LouAnne brought some fast food breakfast for the two of us. Our neighbor, a sheriff's deputy who knew his way around the area, drove LouAnne to the hospital and stopped at the Hardee's across the highway from the hospital. I ate no more than half the chicken biscuit and hash browns that morning. I had no appetite for anything. Lilli was hungry, however, and we ordered some toast, eggs, and mandarin oranges from room service. We memorized that phone number for the hospital kitchen within days.

LouAnne mentioned a cart parked outside Lilli's room.

"What cart?" I asked.

LouAnne said that there was a cart full of these hazmat suit parts and pieces and that she had asked the nurses about them. "We don't have to dress in those outfits, since we're Lilli's family members, but the team has to dress out so they don't spread germs from one patient to another."

Lilli and I told LouAnne what we had learned about leukemia that morning. It was all hypothetical at that point, but I had looked up enough information about leukemia on my phone to hope and pray for ALL instead of AML. The survival rates published online were drastically different for the two main types of pediatric leukemia, and ALL had a much higher rate of survival. I couldn't tell Lilli what I had read, however. Lilli just wanted to get back to school as quickly as possible.

Acute Myeloid Leukemia

Dr. Wofford returned to Lilli's room when she heard that both LouAnne and I were there. Dressed in the hazmat suit this time, she pulled up a chair at the foot of Lilli's bed and began sharing the detailed diagnosis with the three of us. Holding my hand, LouAnne sat on the sofa bed, and I sat in a recliner between her and Lilli's bed. Dr. Wofford proceeded to say that she had taken a look at Lilli's cells under the microscope and that she could confirm that Lilli had AML, Acute Myeloid Leukemia. She told us that this type of leukemia is harder to beat, at which point LouAnne and I squeezed each other's hand as tightly as ever and looked at each other holding back tears. My lips quivered while I tried to hold my emotions in check and had to turn away from Lilli.

Dr. Wofford sensed our emotions and pulled the mask from her face so that we could see her face when she delivered the next part of her message, "From what I know about you, Lilli, I believe that you can fight this." I was encouraged by what Dr. Wofford said and by the directness with which she delivered the message. I also noticed that she didn't say, "you can beat this." She stopped short of that degree of confidence.

Doing a search for "pediatric AML leukemia" turned up lots of information, from academic journal articles to blogs to quackery and everything in between. The information was not reassuring. One of the first hits revealed the pediatric AML survival rates of 65-75%. I couldn't get that number out of my head. Of the 500 children per year diagnosed with AML in the US, this survival rate meant that as many as 175 of those kids would not live five years. Would my LilliBug be in that 175?

I read that AML was one of the two main strains of leukemia, more common in adults, that affected the bone marrow such that myeloid cells, a kind of white blood cell, would take over the bloodstream through the excess creation of baby or immature cells that would crowd out other kinds of blood cells like red cells and platelets. Dr. Wofford had already told us this about AML, but I had already forgotten due to the fog of information overload. These immature white cells called "blasts" are naturally occurring, but a percentage greater than 5% can be a sign of leukemia. Other signs of leukemia are lower platelet counts, lower hemoglobin, and higher white blood counts. Lilli was a textbook case, with all of those signs. On the outside Lilli looked like a very sick girl, and on the inside her blood was malformed due to the cancerous cells' causing the bone marrow to be dumb and unable to differentiate cancerous cells from normal cells.

Dr. Wofford presented us with a printout of the standard-of-care for a pediatric AML patient, the roadmap for treatment they would follow, the same treatment Lilli would receive if she were a patient at Brenner, Duke, Chapel Hill, or any of the other Children's Oncology Group hospitals near us. The roadmap for Lilli consisted of roughly four months of chemotherapy. Each month would consist of 28 days in the hospital, during which time Lilli would have to endure between four and ten days in a row of multiple high dose chemo infusions, followed by two or three days at home before going straight back to the hospital to be admitted for the following round. The chemo treatments were divided up between *induction* rounds, the first few months when the treatments were intended to get Lilli's cancer into remission, and *consolidation* rounds, the later rounds that were to kill any remaining cancer cells that were hiding out.

I understood the general idea for this plan, but I didn't realize how formulaic it was and how well the team could predict the rhythm of Lilli's response to the treatments. Sure, there were unknowns, like how well Lilli's cancerous cells would respond to the chemo or how many infections Lilli might have to fight off during each round, but predictability resulted from decades of research and clinical trials.

The rhythm of each month included a week or so at the beginning when Lilli's bone marrow would still produce blood cells, good or bad, during which time the team would pump IV bags of toxic chemicals into her body. Each time Lilli got a chemo infusion the team dressed up again in their hazmat suits and warned us not to get close to any of the chemo fluids and not to touch Lilli's sweat, spit, or urine during that time.

After those highly toxic drugs were absorbed into Lilli's bloodstream and went to work, Lilli's bone marrow would bottom out and stop producing blood cells. There would be a low point during each round when Lilli's body would have no white blood cells and would only have red blood and platelets as a result of transfusions. It was at those low points when Lilli was most susceptible to infections. Going through those nadirs was scary. Following each one of those valleys would come an increase in Lilli's blood counts, as her bone marrow would reawaken and begin making new cells. We would pray that those new cells would not be cancerous and that Lilli would achieve and maintain remission, which was not a guarantee.

There was a lot of paperwork for us to sign, and the team gave us a few days to review the forms before requiring our signatures. I asked, "What if we don't sign these forms?" and Dr. Wofford responded that they would still provide treatment to Lilli per the standard of care because she was their patient. This took some pressure off me and LouAnne to make decisions about Lilli's care, because otherwise we would have only a few days to become experts in cancer treatment in order to make informed decisions about the treatments. Dr. Wofford told us that Brenner was one of a network of pediatric cancer hospitals, which provided some level of comfort that Lilli would receive the same treatment that doctors from around the country would be administering to other pediatric AML patients. Dr. Wofford added that there were two clinical trials that Lilli could participate in. One was a fairly innocuous trial, which involved our using chlorhexidine antibacterial body wipes on Lilli's body daily, in an effort to reduce the potential for bacterial infections. Lilli didn't mind the prospect of using wipes on her body after bathing each day, and we agreed that we would sign up for that trial. That was the easy decision.

The second trial was more complicated. It involved the standard protocol of chemotherapy drugs plus an additional chemo. Who in the world thinks that a newly-minted cancer parent would know enough to make a critical decision about chemotherapy drugs? If we were to enroll Lilli in this trial, then she would get an additional drug not included in the standard of care. What if this additional drug were the one drug that would actually cure her? What if this additional drug were the one drug that would have major side effects that would kill her? How were we supposed to make this call?

We asked Dr. Wofford for her expert medical opinion about the trial option and the additional chemo that Lilli would receive. She described the technical aspects of the trial, but ultimately, she said that it would be up to us to decide. She also pointed out that if a trial had already proved exceedingly successful, then it would have already become the new standard; conversely, a terribly unsuccessful trial would result in that trial's being stopped in its tracks. I concluded that the benefit Lilli might realize from this extra chemo must not be all that substantial and that we should ask for Lilli's input before making a call on a trial that seemed like a virtual toss-up.

As a 12-year-old, Lilli was now aware of her situation, that she faced potential death as a result of her illness. Had she been a much younger patient, then LouAnne and I would've made all the calls about her treatment plans; instead, we included Lilli in any decisions that impacted her health. We asked Lilli for her thoughts about the trial involving the extra chemotherapy, as she heard everything from Dr. Wofford the same as we did. We didn't have private conversations with the team. We discussed Lilli's treatments in the patient room with Lilli wide awake, an active participant. We decided to sleep on the decision about the trial, as we had a few days before that decision would need to be made.

Ultimately, we decided not to enroll in the trial for the additional chemotherapy. Who knows what impact it could've had on Lilli's outcome, but we didn't look back at that point. There was too much to worry about with the standard AML protocol that we couldn't second guess ourselves.

I didn't eat lunch the day of Lilli's diagnosis. I spent the rest of that day texting and calling my close friends and family to let them know the news. Dad's brother, Richard, called to pray with me over the phone. He started to talk to me but realized that I was speechless. I couldn't talk because whenever I tried to say something I got choked up. I didn't want to break down in front of Lilli, so I remained quiet on the phone while Richard prayed. Dad called to say that he was praying, was there for us, and would help out in whatever way possible. My three older sisters called and texted to let me know they were praying and ready to help out, too. LouAnne and I got many texts and Facebook messages from friends at church who were part of a Facebook group that LouAnne and I updated throughout the previous night. I was overwhelmed by all the support that we got, almost immediately after Lilli was diagnosed.

LouAnne's parents were on the way to our house that evening, and LouAnne decided to spend the second night with Lilli. While we hadn't quite figured out what our long-term plan would be to manage our time in the hospital, LouAnne and I were already modeling what became our plan: alternating nights in the hospital and at home, and spending two nights in a row at home or in the hospital over the weekends. It would be weeks before LouAnne and I would share the same bed again and months until we'd be at home without other family members there to look after our other kids. We agreed to sacrifice our time as husband and wife in the service of our roles as father and mother for as long as it took for Lilli to get better.

Siblings

I had about thirty minutes on the drive home that night to think about how to break the news to Lilli's younger brother and sister. Amelia was in the fourth grade. Collin was in the first grade.

How do I tell our other kids that their sister has cancer? Will Amelia and Collin even understand what this means? I can't lie to them, but can I tell them everything? I'll just have to go with my heart.

I needed the half hour drive to Greensboro to clear my mind, cry the tears that I had been holding in all day, and get in the right frame of mind to share the news. A few days earlier LouAnne and the girls had watched a Hallmark movie about a boy with cancer. I didn't watch the movie with them, but they told me it was about a little boy who died from cancer.

So yes, our kids probably have a clear idea of what cancer could do and that someone could die from cancer.

I had to pick up Collin from the neighbors who had taken him in earlier that day so that he could play with some of his friends and not dwell on his big sister. The neighbors answered the door, looked at me, and absorbed the news that Lilli had leukemia. We all stood there in silence, not knowing what to say. Collin was playing with the neighbors' boys and eating pizza for dinner. While he probably knew that something was up, I waited until we got home to say anything.

Amelia had gone to a friend's house, and the friend's mom drove Amelia home shortly after I picked up Collin and took him home. The mom had the same stunned look on her face when she dropped off Amelia. After the kids were there together I called them into the living room where I asked them to sit down next to me on the ottoman. In as calm a voice I could muster, I told the kids that their sister had to stay longer at the hospital and that she had been diagnosed with leukemia, a kind of blood cancer.

"Will this be Lilli's last Christmas?" Collin asked. He was a first grader and seven years old at the time, but he had some understanding of life and death. Nothing I had ever done in my life had prepared me for the moment my seven-year-old son asked if his sister was going to die, but I instinctively decided to be open and honest with my kids.

"It's possible that Lilli could die, son," I said. "We'll be praying that she lives through this, but the doctors told us that she's very sick." I added, "I don't know what'll happen. It's possible that this will be her last Christmas. We hope that she'll live through this and get better, but there's no guarantee. Her cancer is a hard one to fight, but the doctors say she can fight it."

Satisfied with my answer, Collin said, "Okay, Daddy, so she might not die."

Amelia was pretty quiet through all of this. She went to her room that night to write down her feelings on paper, a very sweet, loving piece of writing from one sister to another.

While asking Amelia and Collin to accept that their big sister might not live to see her next birthday, I was also accepting this potential fate in my own heart. There was no guarantee that Lilli would live to see Christmas 2014, which was just eleven days away. There was no guarantee that Lilli would ever leave the hospital, either. I had to shift from a belief that all my children would outlive me to a new possibility that I might have to bury a child.

Later that evening LouAnne's parents, Joe and Janet, pulled into our driveway. "Papa Joe" was a semi-retired English teacher, and "MaMaMa Janet" was a retired nurse who volunteered at a local pregnancy center. They had enough flexibility in their lives to stay with us for a while. They had packed for a long visit, agreeing to help us as long as necessary, as long as they could go back home to Georgia once a month to pay bills and to check on things around the house. They would be our lifeline for months, allowing me and LouAnne to keep our jobs, work alternating days, and spend alternating nights sleeping at the hospital with Lilli. I walked outside to help them unload their minivan when my next-door neighbors pulled up. Scott, who had heard our news from LouAnne, walked over and put his arm around me. I stood in silence, not able to say a word, and with tears in my eyes. He too was choked up and said that they were there for us if we needed anything.

That night I decided to post something on my personal Facebook page. I chose a picture of Lilli from my phone and posted this: "Our lives changed today. We learned that our precious Lilli has AML Leukemia and is about to begin a months-long battle against cancer. She is a rock." There were lots of responses from friends and family, all well-intentioned and mostly well-received. I had the most trouble reading posts in which folks tried to offer medical advice, suggest that marijuana or essential oils would cure Lilli, share stories about friends who had fought cancer successfully, or quote statistics that were inaccurate or irrelevant to our situation.

The first night at home I couldn't bear to sleep alone in our bedroom with a view down the hall to an open door and Lilli's empty bed. Amelia and Collin were also scared by what might happen to their sister, so the three of us slept together in our king-sized bed. I'm not sure what the sleeping arrangements were on nights when LouAnne slept at home, but for weeks I slept in the same bed as Amelia and Collin, holding on to them tightly as I struggled to fall asleep.

Surgery

....

Lilli was born in a surgical suite, but she had very little experience with surgery or hospitals beyond that. Her tongue was clipped because she had been born tongue-tied, a condition where extra skin under the tongue inhibits the otherwise normal workings of the tongue. Lilli was at risk for having speech impediments from this fairly common medical condition. When Lilli was a toddler, LouAnne and I agreed to have her tongue surgically clipped in an outpatient procedure that was quick and with no lasting side effects, our only experience with pediatric surgery until that Sunday morning in 2014.

On the day of Lilli's diagnosis, the oncology team told us that she would need surgery to insert a central line. There was a leap between a snip of the tongue and a central line. The standard of care for pediatric AML patients involved lots of blood draws and transfusions and the administration of intense chemo via IV.

51

Instead of having an IV through a needle in the arm, Lilli would have a central line surgically connected to her central arteries, a direct connection to her heart. Sunday morning, Lilli was scheduled for that surgery.

It was still dark Sunday morning when I drove back to the hospital, just in time to find the nurses' prepping Lilli for the ride over to the surgical suite. It was a Sunday, and the pediatric surgical clinic was not operational; instead, Lilli would ride through a maze of corridors in the adult wing of the hospital and down a patient elevator to what felt like a dungeon. It was a dark, windowless series of corridors and rooms made of concrete block walls with tile ceilings and humming fluorescent lights. LouAnne and I escorted Lilli into a very small room where we had to fill out some paperwork and sign off on all kinds of possible side effects, including death. It's standard for hospitals to have patients acknowledge that death is a possibility, but this was the first time that we had to do it for Lilli. The only way to save her life was to put her through a series of procedures that could also take her life. I stared at the waiver form, clipboard, and ball point pen for an eternity before I could bring myself to sign the parental waiver.

We kissed Lilli and said that we'd see her back in her room when she finished the procedure. LouAnne and I had to find our way back up and across the building that was a perfect stranger to us two days earlier. We didn't have much to say to each other as we retraced our steps, but we held hands like our daughter's life depended on us. In Lilli's empty room we didn't know what to do with ourselves. Going back and forth between pacing the floor and sitting down to rest, I impatiently waited for the nurses to bring Lilli back to us.

A nurse wheeled Lilli back into the room, and later the surgeon came in to let us know that the procedure had gone well and that the scarring should be minimal. Lilli had an incision near her sternum where a central line exited through that incision and extended out into a two-pronged spaghetti-like appendage, tucked under a sterile dressing that concealed a loop, providing some slack to the lines should they snag on anything outside Lilli's body. Lilli was happy to have the IV removed from her arm, as it had become itchy and annoying, but she was exhausted.

Lilli now had an artificial appendage, and her body and mind had gone through a lot of stress by that time. "LilliBug, let's ask the nurses if you can get out of that gown and put on your own pajamas. Maybe that will help you feel better," LouAnne suggested. Lilli smiled, and the nurse said, "Sure, you can wear whatever you like as long as we can access your lines." LouAnne helped Lilli put on her pajamas, realizing that tops with button fronts or loose necks would work best with these flexible tubes sticking out of her chest.

Dr. Wofford came in to let us know that while Lilli was in surgery for her central line the team went ahead and performed additional procedures. Dr. Wofford performed a bone marrow aspirate to check Lilli's marrow for cancer, did a spinal tap to check for the presence of cancer going to Lilli's brain, and injected Lilli's spinal fluid with chemotherapy. There was a lot to absorb that Sunday, and Dr. Wofford let us know that it would be a day or two before they would start the IV chemotherapy infusions in earnest.

That afternoon, Joe and Janet arrived with Amelia and Collin in tow. After washing up in the vestibule, Amelia and Collin couldn't wait to get in the room with their big sister. Lilli's face lit up when she saw them, and she asked if they could jump in bed with her. "Sure," LouAnne said, "just be careful with her lines." Collin jumped in the bed first to cuddle with his sister, reminding me of all the times he had done the same thing at home. There were several years, when Collin was a preschooler, when we'd awake to find that Collin had walked down the hall and climbed into Lilli's bed in the middle of the night. The two of them would be locked in a bear hug in Lilli's narrow twin bed. The hospital bed wasn't much larger, but the side rails provided extra protection from falling off.

Joe and Janet were not as quick to enter Lilli's room. From the glass in the vestibule door they could see their oldest grandchild in a weakened state. Janet turned her head to hide her tears from Lilli's view and regained her composure before opening the door. LouAnne hugged her parents and encouraged them to come in and cheer up Lilli. Collin and Amelia took turns climbing in bed with Lilli as the room filled up with family members who claimed every seat in the place, took in this new world of pediatric cancer, and made small talk about anything but leukemia.

The doctor on duty the following day was not Dr. Wofford but was instead Dr. Russell, a nice young male doctor who spoke in a matter-of-fact and authoritative manner, "We know that Lilli will require many blood transfusions during her stay in the hospital, and I think that we should go ahead and give her a bag of blood this afternoon. She's anemic, and a blood transfusion will boost her energy level."

A bag of blood? Okay…I guess this is just the kind of jargon they use in the hospital. I've never thought of using that expression ever before in my life, but hey, bring on the bag of blood!

The lab had to type and match Lilli's blood with what was in the blood bank, which took some time, during which LouAnne and I had a chance to review more paperwork about various procedures, including transfusions, and to sign off on those procedures and their side effects, again with the possibility of death resulting from these life-saving procedures. We signed off, taking a little less time to think it through the second time.

The first bag of blood arrived later that afternoon. It was red, like blood red. Hanging on the IV pole, the blood dripped, dripped, dripped into a pump and tubing that connected ultimately to Lilli's central line. I dwelled on those made-for-TV movies where the villain would pump some air into a hospital patient's IV line, causing ultimately a death that would go untraced. An irrational fear, I know, but that fear preoccupied my mind more than I'd like to admit. Other fears included: having mis-matched blood types, a rejection of the cells, a tear in the central line, a bacterial infection from the blood going straight to Lilli's heart, and worse.

Early in Lilli's treatment, we got a visit from Doug, a man from our church who was a survivor of AML leukemia. While his treatment plan was totally different from Lilli's and included a stem cell transplant using his own cells as a source, he comforted Lilli by telling her that he had gone through many of the same things. He told her how his chemo treatments had gone and how he had the same kind of central line surgically inserted in his chest. It also comforted me to know that Doug had fought a similar fight to the one ahead of Lilli and had survived for ten years by the time of Lilli's diagnosis. Doug and his family would continue to comfort us through his prayers and words of encouragement.

Doug provided some comfort to us parents. Lilli's pajamas provided some comfort to her. The room, on the other hand, had yet to be personalized into something comfortable. I started with the white board. This white board on the wall near the door just inside Lilli's room, a standard board that documented Lilli's blood counts on a regular basis, had a happy-face scale for how much pain she was feeling, a place for the name of the doctor and nurse on duty, a place for her blood counts, and a place for comments. I took some ownership of this board by adding a space for counting the number of smiles in a day, the smile-ometer. While the hematology/oncology team concerned themselves with white blood, hemoglobin, and platelet counts, LouAnne and I spent time each day focused on Lilli's emotional health. We tried to take Lilli's mind off things by making jokes and having her brother and sister visit enough to put a smile on Lilli's face. I challenged Lilli to increase her smile count each day, and she got up to a personal daily record of 40 smiles per day.

Meals + Trains

On Sunday night, some of our friends from our Sunday school class at church stopped by to visit and drop off some hospital necessities, like magazines, candy, snacks, and some posters with photos of our friends from church. They asked me and LouAnne to step out into the hallway for a minute, where they hugged us and then handed us an envelope full of money they had collected that morning. I was speechless. I wanted to say something, but my cheeks got hot and my lips twitched as I sensed my emotional breakdown. Instead, I just looked at our friends and nodded my head. I was able to say, "Thank…You," and that was that.

I had no idea what the costs would be for us as cancer parents, but I had already figured out that parking – which was cash only at the time – would eat into our budget by about $10 per day per car. Later we would discover some tricks of experienced 9th floor families who knew which staff member would provide a week-long parking pass, when available, one per family. But that night an envelope of cash meant that we could keep driving to the hospital and park in the maze-like parking deck for a few weeks. We could also pay for some of the cafeteria food or fast food in the area.

Continuing to eat out would've destroyed our family's budget. One of our friends from church asked if we had ever used MealTrain, an online resource for folks in need of meals, usually following health scares, births, or funerals. Would we like to use MealTrain to schedule dinners at our house? If so, would we want folks to bring us dinner every night? Every other night? Weekends? LouAnne and I had a lot to think about. We had decisions to make about Lilli's treatments, but we also had to make sure our other kids could eat. And we couldn't burden my in-laws with cooking on top of everything else they did.

This MealTrain question triggered other questions. Would we start a GoFundMe page for our finances? Would we want to put ourselves out there like that? Would we want others to raise money in Lilli's name? What about t-shirts? What about wristbands? What would we put on those fundraiser items? What about Facebook? What about Instagram? Would we post in a public forum? Would we maintain our privacy and share information with only our friends and family? What about CaringBridge? What about setting up a special bank account for donations? Who would manage the funds? Who would write updates online? Would we call people and give them updates? Would we have time to respond to people's e-mails? Texts? Facebook messages and posts?

The MealTrain option seemed to make a lot of sense, as neither LouAnne nor I would be able to cook all the meals we would need for the four of us who would be at home plus LouAnne's parents, albeit on alternating nights for me and LouAnne. If people in our community were willing to help out and could cook a meal, then why not take advantage of MealTrain? Our friends from church helped set up the page and paid the fee for managing a calendar of meals and posting updates. LouAnne and I decided that the MealTrain site could also be a primary means of sharing updates about Lilli and the rest of our family. I was the designated writer for these updates. We decided, too, that meals on alternating nights would be just fine, as there were generally leftovers for the following day's lunch or supper.

I ate all kinds of meals cooked by members of our community. Chicken. Spaghetti. Lasagna. Pot roast. Chicken pot pie (the best I've ever had). More chicken. Pizza. Barbecue. Stew. Soup. Salads. More chicken. Sandwiches. Pudding. Cake. Cupcakes. Fruit salad. We had more food than if someone had died. In addition to the late afternoon deliveries of dinner through the MealTrain sign-up scheduler, one of my students would deliver a quiche weekly to our front door before we were out of the house for carpool. For certain, we did not starve during Lilli's treatments.

As for Facebook and other social media outlets, I decided to post updates about Lilli on my personal Facebook page, knowing that it would be friends and family who would see those posts. I saved the more detailed updates for MealTrain, e-mailing invitations to that page as people showed interest in providing us with a meal or curiosity about Lilli's condition. I also posted some updates on Instagram as Lilli's friends had been posting there. While our kids didn't have any social media accounts at that time, Lilli had a few friends who were already on Facebook and Instagram.

Back at Lilli's school, the teachers and students were shocked. They began to post to Instagram with the hashtag #LilliStrong. We adopted that same hashtag, and I rediscovered the Instagram account that I had started a few years earlier when I was traveling out of town for academic conferences.

I also found Facebook and CaringBridge to be resources as I sought to read and learn about other patients who were fighting similar illnesses. Early in Lilli's treatment, LouAnne found out about a woman from Greensboro, a wife and mother to young children. She was in the adult cancer wing at the same hospital as Lilli, and I imagined that I could see her room at night as I drove to and from the hospital. This mom had a Facebook page that updated friends and family and others about how she was doing. When Lilli was first diagnosed this mom was pretty far along in her treatment. It seemed like the chemotherapy was not as successful in attacking her cancer, but she had been able to leave the hospital a few times during treatment. There were posts with photos of her with her kids and husband, and there were posts from her community of supporters who were pulling for her. Her CaringBridge page had comments from her young children who posted things like, "We still believe in you, Mom. You've got this."

During December and January, I followed this patient as she got worse and worse. At some point, she posted that the cancer was taking over her body and that the doctors had done everything they could for her. A few days later, her husband posted details of her final days along with information about her funeral and a request for privacy for the family to process their grief. I felt like a voyeur, on one hand, but was appreciative for the story of this young mother, as it helped me contemplate all the possibilities. Watching a family fight cancer while maintaining their faith and dignity gave me some solace that I was not alone in this fight.

What if LouAnne and I have to plan a funeral? Where would I bury a child? Would I push people away and seek privacy and isolation? Or would I invite the world in to see what cancer can do to a child?

Christmas

....

We were determined to make Christmas 2014 special. If this were going to be Lilli's last Christmas, then LouAnne and I wanted to stay as close to our family traditions as possible. If we had been at home, then we would've celebrated the Christmas Eve service with our church family in Greensboro. Our associate pastor asked if Lilli might be up for reading the Christmas story from the Bible to be played over the A/V system at the church for the evening service. Lilli was amenable, so we set up my tripod and camera in room 912, used some of the Christmas decorations from our friends and family as a backdrop near the window seat, and had Lilli wear a shirt that covered up her central line's going out to the IV pole that we kept out of the shot. Though visibly weak, Lilli aced the Christmas reading. Back at home in front of my computer, I played a few Christmas tunes on the low whistle and overlaid those tracks onto Lilli's video.

When Christmas Eve came around our family was in two different places, skyping in to the church service. Amelia and I huddled around my computer in our basement office while LouAnne, Collin, Lilli, and my in-laws huddled around a tablet in the hospital. With sketchy church wi-fi, the connection kept buffering and dropping, but we saw most of the service including Lilli's reading the birth story from Matthew and Luke. After the service, Amelia and I stuffed my car with Christmas presents and drove to Winston-Salem on a spooky, cold, and foggy evening. I needed four trips to carry the load of gifts, even with a hospital cart that I borrowed from the unit to help me haul more stuff at once.

The nurses came around with a few gifts from former patients' families, including an envelope with $100 cash and a letter from the donating family. I struggled to read the note because our experience was still so raw and new and also because this family's story included their son's passing away as an 18-year-old. The letter included a photo of their son sitting in the driver's seat of a classic pick-up truck. The envelope also included a wristband with their son's name on it, again a hard one to swallow when our family was brand new to being a cancer family. What was special about receiving this envelope was that the nurses on the unit were given a handful of these envelopes by the family and were asked to hand them out to patients who were deserving. I wondered if I would ever be that father, that family member who would go back and give back to families in need. I couldn't see it in the short-term, but perhaps I could be that generous further down the road, past the initial shock and emotion of this whole new world.

On Christmas Eve, we opened one gift each, in keeping with our family tradition. LouAnne's parents were there, and they spent a few nights with Amelia and Collin at the Ronald McDonald House (RMH) just up the hill from the hospital so that we could all be together for the Christmas holiday. We spent some time together as a family on Christmas Eve, but we had to split up before going to bed. LouAnne and I shared the room with Lilli, the first time since Lilli's diagnosis that we were in the same town, much less the same room. LouAnne slept on the sofa bed and I the recliner. We crammed Christmas gifts in every nook and cranny of the room so that Lilli could be with us when we all opened our gifts.

Santa Claus somehow knew where to find all three of our kids. We missed Santa's formal visit to the 9th floor because Lilli had been under isolation orders when he came. With his fuzzy costume and beard and moustache he would've been a prime candidate to absorb all kinds of germs from kids' rooms. And the jolly old elf is too big to ask him to don all the hazmat suit trappings to go into patient rooms. He made it back, however, for Christmas Eve. He left a large red sack full of presents in Lilli's room in the middle of the night, and he left a large box full of presents outside the door of the RMH room for Amelia and Collin. The red cotton sack was slammed full of presents for a pre-teen girl, her siblings, and a few presents, like gift cards, for the whole family.

Amelia had been sick for a few days leading up to Christmas, and we weren't sure if the doctors would clear her to visit. On Christmas Eve, however, Amelia started feeling a bit better, and the team cleared her as long as she wore a face mask around Lilli. She and Collin awoke with Joe and Janet at the Ronald McDonald House, and we FaceTimed with them early that morning before they headed over to the hospital. We opened presents for a long time, as there were lots of Christmas presents in a one-person patient room where Lilli was still a patient who had to endure various procedures, vitals, and labs. She had finished the first course of chemo, ten straight days of three different chemo drugs, the day before Christmas, and she was feeling their effects. While her hair had not started to fall out yet, she was losing weight due to appetite loss and feeling some pain in her muscles and joints. We had to take a few breaks while opening presents to pace ourselves according to Lilli's energy levels.

Around New Year's Day, my dad and sisters Tammy, Toni, and Teri came to visit. Dad had some experience with cancer patients, having watched his brother, Anthony, undergo treatment for melanoma in the early 80s and having stayed with my cousin, Stephen, who fought cancer several times. Both of these men in my family passed away at young ages after fighting the cancers that ultimately took their lives. Even with this experience, however, Dad had not seen a grandchild suffer from cancer or anything as life-threatening as what Lilli was fighting. My sisters, too, had some life experiences with hospital rooms, but they had not spent months at a time in the hospital with a child fighting cancer.

As the baby in the family, I had been teased by my older sisters growing up, but my sisters had also been like extra mothers to me, especially after we all lost our mom way too early. I needed my sisters' support, and they all helped in their own ways. They all mobilized their own support networks back at home and had their friends and family prepare care packages, cards, letters, and gift cards to send to Lilli. They stayed a few days near the hospital and visited Lilli and the rest of us at the hospital and in Greensboro.

Around that same time, the hospital instituted a restriction on visitors under 18 years old due to a local flu outbreak. The nurses said that this was common each and every year around the same time. Lilli was devastated. She handled the cancer diagnosis like a rock, but she couldn't take the news that she wouldn't be able to see her little brother and sister for weeks. When Lilli's team got word of the restrictions they told us that at some point they'd be okay if we were to sneak Lilli's siblings up to the room, as they recognized the importance of addressing Lilli's emotional and mental health alongside her physical health.

For weeks, Lilli had to rely on me, LouAnne, and other adult visitors to keep her company. I couldn't wait until the ban was lifted, myself, as it was hard to watch my girl fight cancer and also be depressed from not seeing her siblings. I sent out a request on social media for folks to send Lilli some cards to cheer her up during this time of isolation, and they delivered. In no time, we had enough cards to plaster the walls and personalize the room even more than before.

9th Floor:Round One

The nurses kept telling us that Lilli was the first AML patient they had treated in several years. A few years earlier they had a few AML patients at the same time, but Lilli was their first AML patient in a while. I sensed that we got special treatment because of Lilli's diagnosis. A staffer from the Ronald McDonald House said that they would always have a room for us and our family as long as Lilli was in-patient. While it was nice to have special treatment, I felt like our special treatment was because Lilli had a lower chance of survival than other patients. Not only had we won the cancer lottery without ever buying a ticket, we were getting special treatment for reasons that seemed unbearable, too.

Our friends would ask how we were able to manage, and I wasn't entirely sure. There were enough things to try to tackle in a given day, as it was, and cancer gave us laser focus and a schedule around so much of our daily lives that it was a matter of responding to the cancer and not being in charge of our own existence. LouAnne and I lived parallel lives and rarely saw each other for more than an hour each day. We swapped off each evening during that hour of sharing the news of the day, and one of us would take an extra night in the hospital each weekend. We tried to balance it so that we each got to go to church on alternating weeks and so that we could spend time at home with Amelia and Collin on alternating weekends. There was no time to be tired, but we were all exhausted by the end of the first round of chemo. And while it wasn't a perfect system, swapping off allowed us to share the burden of being pediatric cancer parents. I couldn't imagine how I would've managed this whole process without being able to spend time at the hospital with my daughter, but I imagined that there were parents out there who had to do this to make ends meet. What a blessing it was to have had two careers with the flexibility that allowed us to take care of Lilli.

While Lilli would live in the hospital, Amelia and Collin still had to go to school half an hour away from the hospital. With their grandparents living in our basement, they would have some stability getting ready for school. Amelia and Collin would get to school each day with either myself or LouAnne, when it was our morning to wake up at home, or with the Rider family, neighbors as well as members of our church. Getting home from school each day was a different story, as we relied on one of Amelia's friends' moms to get the kids home. Managing our carpool became a community effort.

Around the time of day when Amelia and Collin would settle in from school, someone from our MealTrain list would deliver dinner for all of us. There would be some small talk about how things were going at the hospital and how we were all coping with things. Then, I would leave to head to the hospital on days when I would spend the night with Lilli. I would arrive at the hospital and park in the parking deck.

This has to be one of the dirtiest parking decks I had ever used. How can a hospital, where germs and cleanliness are of utmost importance inside the building, allow their parking structures to become as filthy as the ones at Wake Forest Baptist?

After a few weeks, I got pretty good at navigating the parking situation, finding the best parking space for access to the main lobby, and circumventing as many hospital visitors as possible to sneak through to the elevator lobby and up to the 9th floor. As an architect, I had always heard complaints about elevator capacity and speed.

"Why didn't you design more elevators?"

"Isn't there some code you have to follow to make sure you have enough elevators?"

"Why did you pick such slow elevators?"

And now I was just like some of my former clients, wishing that there were more elevators and faster elevators so that I could get to Lilli's room as soon as possible. Although I had spare clothes in Lilli's room, inside the wardrobe, I would still have bags full of things that I carried back and forth from home. I would carry mail for Lilli, cards or small packages that people would send to our house, fresh clothes for Lilli, snacks for all of us who stayed overnight, and my laptop computer to get work done when I could. I'd climb in an elevator with all my bags and push the call button for the 9th floor with the back of my hand or elbow. I had learned a few tricks for minimizing my exposure to germs, including trying not to use my hands or fingers to touch door hardware or elevator buttons. The elevators at Brenner drove me crazy in another regard. Their call bells, that I imagined were mellifluous when they were brand new, had become these annoying and horrendous, dull versions of their former selves. They sounded like something out of science fiction sound effects intended to scare more than soothe. In addition to the bells and chirps from the IV poles, this elevator chime is another sound that is burned into my memory.

Exiting the elevator at the 9th floor I'd turn towards the pediatric wing, pass by the hematology-oncology clinic, and go towards the double doors leading to the locked units. Pressing the buzzer, I'd wait on the nurse to unlock the door with the remote button before going through the doors and walk briskly down the hall with the normal pediatric patients while holding my breath so as not to catch anything. Turning the corner towards Lilli's unit, I'd put on my brave face, not knowing what would greet me on the other side of door. There was a niche with a crash cart across the hall from Lilli's room, a constant reminder of the thin line between life and death on this hallway. Occasionally there would be families outside the rooms, collecting themselves or having private discussions. There was limited space there for any kind of discussion, and folks would make do with whatever they had. The consultation room doubled as a family break room with snacks and a microwave and as a library for checking out books and movies, not the place where you'd want to have a sensitive conversation.

Walking through the solid door of room 912, I'd enter the vestibule where I'd have to wash up, trying to sanitize my hands and forearms enough that I wouldn't give Lilli any of the germs from outside. At the same time, however, I wondered about my shoes and what kinds of germs they probably carried from the parking deck. From the vestibule I could look in on Lilli and LouAnne and assess their moods before going into the room.

Life on the 9th floor was mostly confined to Lilli's patient room. For the first month Lilli was isolated because of the unknown virus or bug that had made her so sick in the first place. In addition to the cancer, Lilli was also fighting something that never revealed itself in the blood cultures. Lilli wasn't allowed to leave her room for weeks, including Christmas and New Year's. She remained in pretty good spirits considering her life was limited to a bed, a sofa, a recliner, a guest chair, a bathroom, a view to the Harris Teeter strip mall and surrounding neighborhood, a view to the helipad atop the parking deck, and cable TV.

When Lilli was a baby and toddler, and up to the age of two, she was our only child. I got to know her quite well as a small child. But as soon as Amelia was born the time I had to spend with Lilli was essentially cut in half. And when Collin was born three years later the distance between me and Lilli (all my children for that matter) grew. I was busy at work. There were more demands on my time. And Lilli, being the oldest, was given more independence and freedom, which also resulted in less parenting on my part. The siblings became very close, and Lilli was the glue holding Amelia and Collin together.

And now it might be one of our other kids who saves Lilli's life. They just had their blood drawn in the 9th floor oncology clinic, and LouAnne said that they did great. I

71

bet it'll be Collin who's the match if one of them is. He and Lilli are very close, and he's her "bud." But it's possible that both or neither of them are matches, too.

Being forced to spend alternating nights in a hospital room with my 12-year-old daughter meant that I got to know this awesome girl all over again. What a gift I had been given! I wished so much that it would not have taken a life-threatening illness to bring me closer to my daughter, but if there were going to be one positive out of this experience it would be that I'd learn more about Lilli, her hobbies, her favorite music, her favorite TV shows, what she liked about school, her quirks, and her spirit all over again.

Spending this much time together inside an acute life-sustaining environment also meant that I had to take care of some things that I would rather not have done, like assisting Lilli when she had to go to the bathroom, take a bath, apply cleansing pads all over her body, and shave her head, as well as being there to clean up things like vomit. No father should have to see his child go through the kind of side effects that cancer treatments rain down on the body.

Taking the good with the bad meant that in between the infrequent throwing up I learned that Lilli and I could bond over HGTV and all the shows about fixing up and flipping houses. As an architect and interior designer, I appreciated the design process and technical side of those shows. Lilli got absorbed into the design process, as well, and the personalities of the hosts. I also learned that Lilli could watch Disney on TV, but only after the little kid shows went off the air in the middle of the day, and that she could tolerate sports. We watched my alma mater's Yellow Jacket football team win the Orange Bowl that year from the hospital room on New Year's Eve, one of the last big wins they've had in recent years.

Lilli spent a lot of time working on arts and crafts. I learned that Lilli is a wizard at arm knitting and other kinds of knitting. When I shared with friends and family how much she enjoyed using yarn of all colors and that she could spend hours on end knitting scarves, we were overwhelmed with all kinds of yarn. Lilli also mastered the art of making bracelets out of rubber bands, using small plastic tools, and she even taught me how to make bracelets like those. When not knitting or making things, Lilli spent lots of time fixing her dolls' hair. While Lilli's hair was falling out, she became a master hair dresser to her dolls.

Team Jerseys

∙∙

We didn't spend much time outside Lilli's room hanging out on the unit. The unit was on the same floor as other pediatric patient rooms, the kind of rooms that might have a kid with a broken leg or appendectomy. Visitors, including us, would have to pass those other patient rooms to get back to the hematology/oncology unit. Once on the unit most patients stayed in their rooms. Some patients would leave their doors open, but most doors were closed, leaving me to wonder who might be behind the doors and what kind of cancer their child had.

The nurses' station formed the core of the unit, around which all the traffic and activity flowed. When Lilli was well and able to get out of her room and walk, we did laps around the nurses' station, passing patient rooms, down the hall past closed office doors, and back around for one lap. Occasionally we would pass or bump into other patients, similarly frail, bald, and trying to get their own exercise. For some patients, their particular chemotherapy regimens would cause them to lose the ability to walk. Those patients would be the ones being pushed around by relatives or friends or going through physical therapy.

A bald little girl whose energy bubbled to the surface in spite of her frailties would hang out at the nurses' station while her single mom went to work. This girl of four or five years would pretend to do work at the desk while coloring in coloring books from the family break room. Lilli and I bumped into her a few times when doing laps around the unit. One morning I awoke early and pulled the chains to raise the window shades. I looked out our picture window to find that this girl's mom had parked atop the deck, usually empty at that time of day. Before leaving for work the mom had written the girl's name in huge letters in the empty parking spaces using her foot to dig into the snow that had fallen the night before. Bundled up and standing outside her minivan in the cold air, this mom waved her arms and screamed out with foggy breath in the direction of the 9th floor, yelling out and miming, "I love you."

LouAnne found out a few years later that this girl did not survive her recurring battle against cancer.

Most families who stayed on the unit would be decked out in t-shirts with their child's name and some kind of quote or bible verse. With words like *Strong, Fight, Army,* or *Team,* t-shirts are one currency for cancer families to pay the bills. A few childhood friends asked if they could organize t-shirt fundraisers for our family, and one of my best childhood friends, Karen, offered to make our first batch of shirts. She had invested in some equipment to make shirts and wanted to help us. I had imagined my children's names on shirts, like soccer uniforms, basketball uniforms, and high school class t-shirts. I had not dreamed about seeing my daughter's name on a shirt for cancer fundraising.

"#LilliStrong." That's what we put on the shirts. We borrowed the slogan from Lilli's friends from school, as they started writing it on their arms and legs with Sharpies when they found out that Lilli had cancer. We agreed to let Karen make t-shirts, and Karen and our friends from church agreed to manage the sales of the shirts. We also allowed the school to organize a sale of wristbands with owls and *#LilliStrong* written on them. Both the t-shirts and the wristbands provided funding that helped us stay afloat financially during the hardest times when Lilli was inpatient.

One morning, the nurse Julie came in to do her initial check-in with us, shortly after she arrived for her 7:00 shift, and she said, "They'll probably be sending you home in the next day or two."

"Oh, really?" I replied, "Why is that?"

"Well, her ANC is coming up. It's 50 today."

I didn't know what Julie was talking about. "What's an ANC?" I asked.

"Absolute Neutrophil Count," she said. "It's part of her White Blood Count."

While I had been vaguely aware of the importance of Lilli's blood counts, up to that point I had not known enough to ask the team for specific blood counts on a regular basis. I looked to the team for general comments about Lilli's condition but didn't realize that I could've known what her counts were daily.

What did she say, again? ANC? Why hasn't anyone told us about this until now? How do they know it'll keep going up? Should we have taken note of this? Should I have been asking for this number all along? Would they have told me? What else aren't they telling us? Are they keeping it a secret? Would I be better off not knowing these numbers but instead just asking about how Lilli's doing generally?

This was the first day I took note of Lilli's blood counts, and from then on, I couldn't go a day without asking how Lilli's counts were. The team would draw blood daily through her central line and test the blood in the lab for white blood, hemoglobin, and platelets, at a minimum. They would generally do a manual differential or "manual diff" of her cells under a microscope to count the different types of white blood cells, like neutrophils, basophils, lymphocytes, monocytes, and others. While I learned that doctors and scientists still don't know what some of these cells types do, specifically, they understand that neutrophils are key to fighting off infections.

The ANC number would play a huge role in my anxiety and mental state from that day forward. Lilli's ANC did continue on an upward trajectory. As her white blood count increased, the ANC increased accordingly. When the team saw the upward trend in her counts they told us Lilli would be discharged. We had lived in the hospital for just under 28 days, and I was amazed at how precisely they had mapped out the treatment. It started with 10 straight days of intense chemo followed by 2.5 weeks of recovery. Lilli's recovery came right on schedule, including her ANC.

This really is a science! Down to the day!

We had not only slept at the hospital for a month, but we had settled into the room and made it our home. There were clothes, hangers, bins full of arts and crafts, blankets, pillows, snacks, drinks, decorations, framed pictures, greeting cards and posters taped all over the room, and toiletries.

It's going to take a moving truck and six trips down to the parking deck before we'll get Lilli out of here.

The job of packing and moving fell on me, the dad, and I got to work as soon as it was clear that they were going to let Lilli go the next day, as long as her ANC was still going up at the appropriate rate.

Lilli left the hospital and was in the outside world for the first time in a month. She had to wear an industrial-looking face mask on the way out of the hospital and anytime she wasn't at home or in her hospital room.

I hope people don't stare at her. She hasn't lost all her hair yet, so it's not clear that she's a cancer patient. They'd be amazed if they knew everything she's been through the last month, but I'm not about to stop and talk to anybody. Let's get out of here as quickly as possible and avoid getting close to anybody. It's flu season, after all.

We rode in two cars from Winston to Greensboro. Lilli hadn't seen the skyline of Winston since the dark, cold night back in December when she and I drove to the emergency room. I pointed out the tall Wachovia Tower to Lilli and asked, "Doesn't it look like it got chopped down and is missing about 15-20 floors somewhere in the middle?" "Ok," Lilli replied, with no interest in architecture that day. She just wanted to get home and see what happened since the night she was last there. I could barely contain my joy to still have my LilliBug, but I was also scared that something could happen to her while we were at home.

Do they really trust us with our daughter while she's going through all these cancer treatments? She still has that central line sticking out of her chest, and they expect us to flush out the two tubes dangling out there. One mistake, and we could cause Lilli to be infected. What if Lilli survives the cancer, only to have her Dad mess up flushing her lines, give her some blood infection, and die from a foolish mistake?

Lilli saw for the first time the three Moravian star lights hanging on our front porch, evenly spaced in place of our regular porch lights. Some friends from church and our next-door neighbor Scott put up the lights a week before Christmas, and Lilli asked us to keep them up until she finished all her chemo. We kept a low profile while Lilli was home. There were a few visitors who brought us dinners; otherwise, we tried to cherish the precious few days that we had together. Lilli was able to sleep in her bed again for the first time in a month, and we had made it past the first of four cycles of chemo.

I started teaching my spring semester design studio while Lilli was at home in January 2015. Around a large conference table one morning I sat down with my fourth-year interior architecture students and said, "You might've heard over the break that my twelve-year-old daughter was diagnosed with cancer." Students gasped at the news, and some of them wiped tears from their cheeks. "Some of you might have experience with cancer, so you know what's going on with my family," I added. Students were speechless as I described some of the details of Lilli's treatments and the impacts they could have on me and my ability to teach.

Continuing to teach full-time provided a psychological outlet away from the hospital and, more importantly, continuity in our family's health insurance.

Precautions

During each month-long round of chemo, Lilli's blood counts would drop as the chemo zapped her bone marrow's ability to make blood cells. During those days when her blood counts zeroed out, there would be many red blood and platelet transfusions. There would not be, however, white blood transfusions nor white blood cell boosting from a drug like Neupogen. With a white blood count of zero Lilli would be at risk for catching anything and everything; therefore, we had to be cautious about our own exposure and cleanliness. I carried multiple bottles of hand sanitizer, washed my hands frequently, and avoided anyone who sneezed, coughed, or looked even the slightest bit sick. I got pretty good at avoiding crowded elevators and at guessing strangers' healthiness from quick glances in hallways, lobbies, and parking decks.

This person looks ill. Thanks, but no, I'll skip this elevator and catch the next one. Oh, I'm waiting on someone. You go ahead. I'll get the next one.

We also had to be careful not to get too close to Lilli. Imagine not being able to hug or kiss your child for weeks or months at a time. That was my life. Of our two daughters, Lilli was the one who showed her affections most publicly and regularly. Lilli was the daughter who sat in my lap until the year she was diagnosed with cancer. She was the *Daddy's Girl* who would hug me and kiss me without any concern for who saw it. I had to accept a new reality that she couldn't kiss anyone and had to keep her distance when hugging. We occasionally stretched the rules by allowing her to sit in my lap in the hospital; however, I went months without kissing my LilliBug. I couldn't risk one of my kisses' infecting her with something I picked up outside her hospital room. We couldn't hug Lilli, and she couldn't hug others, either. This was particularly hard for me to witness, as Lilli loved to hug younger kids. If you had seen Lilli at church before she was diagnosed with leukemia, you would've witnessed a sweet little girl who encouraged and loved other children and showed her love through hugs.

She didn't get that behavior from me, that's for sure. I love people, and all, but I'm pretty shy around folks and am not one to run up and hug people.

Food was another risk. Given the possibility of contracting an infection or virus from unwashed or mishandled produce, Lilli couldn't eat fresh fruits or vegetables, which bothered her for a long time. Both she and Amelia would clean their plates at dinnertime. Fruits, vegetables, and salads were some of Lilli's favorites. She could do without junk food, but she really missed her salads. There were other dietary restrictions on things like raw honey, soft cheeses, and other foods that were healthy but prepared in such ways as to be unsafe for an immune-compromised person like Lilli.

My challenge as a Dad was to find foods that Lilli could eat and ones that she wanted to eat. The oncology team said they would support any calories she could get in her body, as long as they met the strict dietary restrictions, as Lilli's low appetite would make it difficult for her to maintain her weight. At first Lilli wanted to eat potato chips, and we bought her all kinds of potato chips. Within a few days her taste buds changed again, and she hated potato chips. We were stuck with loads of chips that Lilli didn't want and the rest of us ate. Later, Lilli fell in love with a cheddar broccoli soup from Panera, and I would run to the Panera across the street from the hospital for soup nearly every day. Later, Lilli's appetite demanded Zaxby's chicken tenders. Without a Zaxby's near the hospital, I'd have to pick up the chicken from a nearby town on the way to the hospital on days when I spent the night. Lilli also had an off and on love affair with Starbucks hot chocolate. I would get the largest hot chocolate they served to get as many calories as possible into Lilli's body. She wasn't gaining weight, but we managed to keep her from losing so much weight that the team would've inserted a feeding tube.

Lilli's restrictions also meant that we started wiping down things at home more and using more hand sanitizer. Lilli became more vigilant around strangers and in public places. She carried around packs of hand wipes and bottles of hand sanitizer, and she avoided crowds. We would skip elevators if they were crowded and would wait on empty elevator cabs when possible. I stopped grabbing door knobs by my hands when possible and started using my wrists to push elevator buttons. I became skilled at using my shirt sleeves as gloves. I had gained a new appreciation for cleanliness and freaked out when I noticed something unclean in any of Lilli's care.

Wishing

It was a cool morning in January 2015 when I drove to Raleigh to chaperone Amelia's 4th grade field trip to the state capitol. I had worked in downtown Raleigh for about four years when LouAnne and I first moved to North Carolina in the fall of 2000, and I would normally look forward to returning to my stomping grounds of Fayetteville Street, which had regained some life after planners tore up the pedestrian mall that had killed it by the time I worked there. I used to walk from my office on Fayetteville Street's pedestrian mall up to the legislative building for lunch in the basement cafeteria, not because of the food but because of the economical prices and the opportunity to eat with a musical genius and friend, Patrick Sky, who worked near there.

But that morning marked Lilli's first return to the children's hospital for the second round of chemo and some tests to see how the first round had worked. It had become clearer to me that some patients responded well to treatment and some didn't. I couldn't take my mind off Lilli and how the tests would go that day. There was no time for nostalgia. LouAnne and her parents had taken Lilli early that morning to the hospital for another bone marrow aspirate, a test requiring that Lilli be put to sleep while they took a small sample of bone marrow from her hip bone, a lumbar puncture, and the beginning of the second course of chemotherapy.

I watched a small group of girls including Amelia and her close friends. The Raleigh field trip was a standard one for elementary schoolers: visit the state legislature and hear about how laws are made in the state, walk through the historic state capitol building, eat lunch in the plaza outside the state history museum, and run around the natural science museum. Before we had gotten very far into that itinerary, I got a call from LouAnne. She was waiting on test results, still, but she had spoken with the social worker.

What LouAnne said shook me to my core. She told me that the social worker was going to recommend Lilli for the Make-A-Wish program. My mind immediately jumped to the conclusion that the hematology-oncology team had determined that Lilli wouldn't make it, that she was near death. I hadn't done any research about Make-A-Wish, but I had visions of sickly children on their death beds making wishes that were granted as a way to make their final weeks on earth fun, memorable, and worth living.

I guess this is it. Lilli's days on earth must be numbered if they're offering to grant her a wish.

I couldn't go anywhere to be alone with my thoughts. I was standing on the sidewalk outside the state legislature, trying to keep my eyes on a handful of 4th grade girls, and I had to keep my composure after just finding out—at least I thought—that my daughter was near death.

Before going into the legislature building I had to wrap up the phone call. I didn't share my fears with LouAnne, but I asked her why the social worker was submitting Lilli's name to Make-A-Wish. "I think it's because Lilli has AML, which is more aggressive," LouAnne said, "and I think that all their AML patients get submitted to Make-A-Wish." This left me wondering whether it was standard protocol for the hospital to send all AML patients forward to Make-A-Wish or if there was something particularly life-threatening about Lilli's case that afforded her special treatment. Either way, this question weighed on my mind throughout the day.

I don't recall what I learned about state government that day. My mind was elsewhere. The North Carolina legislature building is an impressive piece of architecture by Edward Durell Stone, and I was interested in the design of the building, inside and out; however, I couldn't appreciate the architecture fully because my mind kept coming back to the notion that my daughter's days were numbered. I went through the motions of the field trip and succeeded in keeping track of these girls while maintaining my composure. Amelia had no idea that I was consumed by the thought that her sister was going to die.

After my peanut butter and jelly sandwich paper bag lunch, we checked out the North Carolina Natural History Museum, a project to which my previous architecture firm had contributed. In the museum, it was a free-for-all in an exciting space for kids to explore. My group of girls ran around from exhibit to exhibit, and we were near the weather exhibit when the phone rang again.

LouAnne called and asked if I could talk. It was hard for me to hear with all the commotion of the museum in the background, but I wanted to hear any updates from LouAnne. She had some results to share with me. "The bone marrow aspirate was very good," she said. "The doctors said that it appears as though Lilli's cancer is in remission and that her body has responded very well to the chemo." That's excellent news, I thought, my mind wandering back to my earlier thoughts about Make-A-Wish.

Maybe it's possible to be granted a wish and still live to see another day. How can I reconcile these mixed messages, though?

The team also told LouAnne that Lilli's siblings were not bone marrow matches for Lilli. We didn't get more details, and we didn't press the issue, either, to learn if Amelia and Collin were matches for each other or not. Of all the news we received that day, this was the worst, even worse than Make-A-Wish's death sentence. I wondered if the oncology team decided to hold onto this bit of news until they could balance it with some better news, like that of Lilli's being in or near remission.

We understood going into the process that siblings have a one-in-four chance of being a match. Children get half their DNA from one parent and half from the other parent. I vaguely recalled some of this genetics from high school biology class, when we did some genetic trait diagrams to predict the chances that our children would have brown hair, blue eyes, or other genetic traits. Each sibling, therefore, would have a one-in-four chance of being a match for another sibling. Had either Amelia or Collin been a match, then the team would've proposed that Lilli go in for a bone marrow transplant at the end of the fourth course of chemo or sooner. Without a sibling match, then Lilli would be in for the entire four courses of chemo. I interpreted this as a hold-your-breath approach to treatment. The oncology team would play the numbers game, obviously, which I took to mean that the sibling matching transplant must have a higher rate of survival than the chemotherapy alone. Lilli's likelihood of survival had gone down with those test results.

Genetics and statistics provided a logical answer to the question, "why couldn't one of her siblings be a match?" It's a one-in-four crap shoot. Two siblings didn't give her a 50% chance; it gave her a 25% chance, twice. Still, I know others who have gone through the bone marrow transplant process who have a sibling who is a match or even multiple siblings who are all matches. This was not our fate.

Without the possibility of a sibling match, I for a split second wondered, "What if we were to have another baby?" Already in our forties, however, LouAnne and I had decided years earlier that we were finished having children. We would have to hope and pray that the standard-of-care chemotherapy regimen would work and that it would kill all the cancer cells. We also understood that the AML leukemia cells in children are more difficult to kill with chemotherapy alone.

When I got back to the hospital that evening and swapped off with LouAnne, I focused on the positive news of the day with Lilli. On the bright side, we learned that Lilli's body responded well to the chemo and that it appeared that her cancer was in remission. It was great to hear the R word this early on in her treatment. The doctors said that most AML patients wouldn't show signs of remission until after the second or third courses of chemo.

I asked Lilli what she would do with a wish from Make-A-Wish. She thought about it all night. We kicked around a few ideas like meeting a favorite TV actress, going to a place like Disney World, meeting a famous musician, or similar things. Ultimately, Lilli said that she'd like to go to Florida to visit her cousins Tyler and Lydia. Wow! I couldn't believe that a 12-year-old would choose a humble request that amounted to a normal family vacation. We would have to wait for several months to find out if Make-A-Wish Central and Western Carolinas would accept Lilli's application and award our family a vacation. We'd have to wait even longer to find out if Lilli's leukemia could be defeated by chemo alone.

Schoolwork

Lilli was worried about missing school from the first minute we checked into the emergency room. The hospital provided one-on-one instruction for pediatric patients, but to participate in the program we would have to withdraw Lilli from Guilford County Schools and enroll her in Winston-Salem Forsyth County Schools. The first week Lilli was in the hospital a teacher came around in hazmat gear to let us know about the hospital school program and to inform us of the enrollment policies. More paperwork.

What? We have to withdraw her from the top-ranked middle school in North Carolina? Lilli worked hard in elementary school and aced all kinds of tests to get into this school. Now we're being asked to withdraw her? Not so fast!

"What if the school system decides to take her magnet school spot as soon as we withdraw her, LouAnne?!" I asked. "There's no guarantee that they won't do that. I wouldn't put it past them, as it would be a strain on the school to hold Lilli's spot."

I needed some reassurance from the school administration that they wouldn't take Lilli's spot. As a middle school focused on academic excellence, a school that is highly selective based on student grades and test scores, it would have a waiting list a mile long of other 6th graders in the county who would love to have that empty seat.

If they take away Lilli's seat in that school, then I'll go to all the local news channels. Who wants to be the principal or superintendent to kick out the cancer kid?

Here was an opportunity for the principal to show her true colors. I emailed the principal Ms. Mott to ask what would happen if we were to withdraw Lilli from Brown Summit Middle School. Would she hold Lilli's spot? And could she put that in writing? Ms. Mott agreed to hold Lilli's place and said that it would be waiting for her whenever she was able to return to school. She put it in writing, on official letterhead, signed the letter, and put our fears to bed. We could then follow through with the process of formally withdrawing Lilli from one county school system and enrolling her in another.

It made Lilli's day—no, her whole week—to be able to work with a teacher one-on-one in the hospital. She had to wait a little while to begin classes, as it was around the Christmas and New Year holidays by the time we worked out all the details. Once the holiday break was over and the middle school teacher, Jamie, was back on the job, he met with us to discuss a plan for teaching Lilli and for communicating with her school.

We couldn't have asked for a better teacher for Lilli than Jamie. He had a grasp of all the subjects Lilli was studying, including the advanced math and language arts, and he had a warmth and humor about him that made it easy for Lilli to connect with him. Jamie would knock on the door around 10:00 or 11:00 each weekday morning, with a smile on his face, and would ask, "Is Miss Lilli ready to work with me this morning?" Left to her own devices, Lilli would sleep all day and do schoolwork at night, but Jamie was on a nine-to-five teaching schedule. He and another teacher had a classroom down the hall for patients who were well enough to get up and out of their rooms, but Jamie always worked with Lilli in her room, with Lilli sitting up in her bed, adjusted so that she could use her rolling over-bed tray as a desk.

Lilli devoured the math problems, as math was her comfort zone and came easily in sixth grade. She struggled to focus on anything that required a lot of reading, like her Language Arts and Social Studies classes. Jamie stayed in touch with her teachers at Brown Summit by email, and he pushed Lilli to work on all of her subjects. I was amazed that Lilli was able to do any work while she was being pumped with toxic chemicals and was at her lowest, with no immune system. But Lilli had enough energy to work with Jamie for about an hour each morning, except when there were holidays or when Lilli was feeling especially low.

The school's counselor Ms. Denny emailed me to ask for Lilli's favorite songs. Lilli was not a fan of many pop stars or singers; instead, she was in the habit of listening to some of the Christian radio stations with LouAnne. Lilli's response to Ms. Denny was that she liked Katy Perry's *Firework* best. I was suspicious of the question in the first place and wondered why the school would ask about Lilli's favorites. Did they have something up their sleeves?

In early February 2015, Lilli was gifted with a video that Brown Summit Middle School produced using *Firework* for background music. The video was choreographed in such a way as to follow Lilli's friends, teachers, staff, and students through the different wings of the school. The video, posted on YouTube, begins with Principal Mott exclaiming, "Ugh! I need a happy pill…Hit it, Tina!" As the music kicks in, the camera leaves the principal's office and heads down the hall, revealing a hallway full of students and staff.

On the day of filming, most students and staff wore blue and purple, Lilli's favorite colors, screamed, yelled, and waved homemade signs decorated with #LilliStrong, owls, and inspiring quotes. The video closed with a scene from the gymnasium, with the whole school singing, "Lilli, you're a firework. Come on show them what you're worth," and yelling, "We miss you, Lilli!" In this video, I witnessed a school that cared about our daughter, friends who danced, sang, and yelled with abandon, not worrying about how they looked to others. This was a special school, and the principal and her staff had won my heart.

The counselor e-mailed me the link to the video, which I shared immediately with Lilli as she lay in her hospital bed. We watched it together then and there. My eyes welled up with tears, and Lilli had a huge grin on her face. She made sure to share the video with Marcia, the self-proclaimed (and rightfully so) "best nursing assistant in the world." Marcia's eyes also teared up as she said, "Lilli, why did you have to make me cry today?" I still watch that video from time to time when I'm looking for a pick-me-up and for proof that there's still good in this world. A quick YouTube search for "#LilliStrong Brown Summit" will turn up this video for anyone else who wants to watch it.

High Cholesterol

I had already scheduled my 2015 annual physical a year in advance, and I fasted, as required, the night before and showed up for the blood work that morning in February. I recalled the time, years earlier, when I had blood drawn for a marriage license when I was a student a Georgia Tech. I went to the campus infirmary for a blood draw, walked back up the hill to the Architecture building, got in the elevator in the basement near the woodshop, and passed out by the time I got to the third-floor studio. Another student found me in the elevator and helped me get to the studio. My instructor made sure that someone ran and got me a bottle of orange juice. From that moment, I was concerned about having my blood drawn. Not only did I dislike the sight of blood but I also found myself drained to the point of passing out when having my blood drawn.

I didn't faint that morning in early 2015, thank God. After the labs that day, I met with my primary care physician who looked me over and talked about my general health. I was having trouble with high blood pressure and being overweight, so he asked me to come back a week later for a blood pressure check with the nurse.

The following day I was at home when I got a call from the nurse who asked if I had actually fasted before coming in for the blood draw. I sat down on the side of the bed and braced myself for whatever was coming. "Certainly, I fasted. I had a little water that morning, but I didn't eat anything after around 11:00 the night before."

"Well, from the numbers on your triglycerides and cholesterol, it looks like you ate a double cheeseburger on the way to the lab."

Ouch! That stings! Does she use that line on a lot of patients?

"The doctor wants to start you on some medication and draw labs again in a few months to see if these numbers improve. We're calling in the prescription, and you can pick it up later today."

This was the wake-up call that I had been waiting for my whole adult life. I didn't act on it immediately, as it had a delayed reaction, but the thought that stuck with me from that day was: What if I watch my daughter fight this hard to save her life and I'm not alive to see her on the other side of leukemia?

I had been athletic as a young boy and teenager. I grew up in rural Putnam County, Georgia, where I could run around and play outside all day without seeing more than my immediate family and a handful of neighbors, the mailman, and the milk truck driver. Although I had video games and Georgia Public Television to tie me to the couch, I got out and played a lot of basketball by myself, hit tennis balls against our concrete block chimney and side of the house, and did the same with a soccer ball. I was physically fit back then.

I played high school basketball, tennis, and golf, and was in great shape until I went to college to study architecture, jokingly referred to as *archi-torture* by others at Georgia Tech. The studio culture was one of pulling all-nighters and working one's fingers to the bone to create striking designs. I fell right into this studio culture and excelled in it, occasionally sleeping at or on my drawing table and generally returning to my dorm room after midnight, not from partying but from working late in the studio to work on drawings and models.

I carried that work ethic into graduate school and into my first job out of school with Michael Graves, my thesis advisor who was a world-renowned architect and product designer. Most people recognize his name from the line of home goods for Target stores that the product design side of the firm started designing when I worked for him in the late 1990s. I enjoyed working in the office because of the prominent projects on which I worked, including an addition to the U.S. District Court in Washington, DC, the court that most people consider the second highest court in the land. When I was working on that addition, the Clinton-Lewinski grand jury was convened in the existing courthouse under Judge Norma Holloway Johnson, one of the judges who provided feedback on our design. I was working on high profile architectural projects at Graves' office, but I was also working ridiculous hours, as many as 80-100 hours a week. I would go to work in the morning, return home for dinner with LouAnne, and then go back to work after dinner and work until around midnight.

I continued this work ethic when LouAnne and I moved to North Carolina and I took a job with a downtown Raleigh architecture and interiors firm. We moved back South after my Mom passed away, to be closer to family and to have a slower pace of life. We accomplished the goal of being closer to home, but the pace of life was still the same. I had worked myself to the point of exhaustion. I was coming home from work, going to bed early at night, and taking long naps every weekend. "My dad naps all the time," one of the kids wrote on a homework assignment designed to learn more about students' families.

With my high blood pressure, high triglycerides, and high cholesterol, I decided that I would make some lifestyle changes as soon as I could, but it would be months before I was hit upside the head by another alarming number. I told Lilli later that day that my arm hurt from having my blood drawn that morning. Without skipping a beat, she said in a deadpan voice, "Daddy, I have my blood drawn EVERY day," with a roll of her eyes and a grin. I had to put another mark on the white board's smile-ometer for that one.

The pills that I picked up from the pharmacy that afternoon included some large gelatinous yellow ones that contained Omega-3 fish oils, supposed to help with my cholesterol and triglycerides, and some small white ones to lower my blood pressure. I went to the small bathroom that Lilli shared with me and LouAnne, poured a small cup of tap water, and looked at myself in the mirror as I took the first dose of these pills that were going to help me live longer.

Dang! Am I going to be "that guy" who relies on drugs to live? Is this the beginning of a life-long reliance on pills? Am I really that bad off that it's too late to undo all the harm that I've done to my body over the years?

I had established a modest presence on Instagram to keep some of Lilli's friends updated on Lilli's progress, but I realized that there was a whole world of Instagram users with similar interests to mine. As I began to worry about my health and how to lose weight I sought out resources for yoga, something that I had practiced years earlier to recover from back surgery.

When we first moved to Greensboro in 2010 I ruptured a disc in my lower back by trying to pick up furniture, boxes of books and magazines, and anything else that weighed a ton. I tried physical therapy, traction, pain pills, steroid injections, and rest. When all that failed, I went with surgery. Dr. G, the surgeon who would perform the discectomy-laminectomy, said that I was the typical candidate for this kind of surgery resulting from a ruptured disc. He said, "It's usually men of your age who are out of shape but think that they're still strong enough to lift heavy objects without having good core strength." He invited the whole family in for a consultation to explain the procedure. As the six of us squeezed into a small exam room in a near empty clinic building one weekend, Dr. G described the surgical procedure as he pointed to my x-rays and MRI results and a plastic model of a spine. I nearly passed out. He asked me to have a seat and let Collin sit in my lap so that I wouldn't collapse. A few days later the surgery went off without a hitch, and I was back home within 24 hours. After the incision healed, I started a regular physical therapy regimen at the orthopedics office. The therapy, designed to develop my core, was a mix of strength training and yoga.

When LouAnne found out that Collin's preschool dance teacher Debbie was starting a parents' yoga class at the school, she made sure that I signed up for it. I was the only man in the class, but the class was small and intimate and easy enough that I could fit in. I had done yoga with Miss Debbie for a few years, off and on, before Lilli got sick. After she got sick and was in the hospital, I had limited time to do yoga in any kind of organized class, which by that time had moved from the preschool to Debbie's house. I made it to a few classes at Debbie's house, but my yoga time was cut short when I started spending every other night in the hospital.

Instagram and Facebook were invaluable sources of yoga inspiration and instruction. They introduced me to such things as monthly yoga challenges. While I realized that they were mostly ways to advertise products and to increase followers for the sponsors and yogis, I decided to join in some yoga challenges following the encouragement from Cindy, a fitness coach and yogi from the west coast. She hosted a group of students virtually through Facebook and Instagram. I benefitted from the monthly yoga challenges, as they held me accountable to practicing yoga every day. I discovered a new use for my old tripod, as I would set up a tripod with a smart phone adapter and take pictures of my yoga poses with my phone.

I started to get in better shape from the yoga. I found that I got better at handling the overnight stays in the hospital where I'd alternate between sleeping in the recliner and sleeping on the sofa bed. Either one of those would do a number on my back by making me stiff, but I couldn't complain about my pain when my daughter was suffering some of the worst pain of her life. I supplemented the yoga practice with an occasional workout from a video series. I didn't lose much weight in the process, but I felt better and had the tools at my disposal when I finally became more motivated to get into shape.

Church

When we decided to move to Greensboro in 2010, LouAnne and I took a leap of faith that I would be in the right profession, moving from full-time architect to full-time professor, that LouAnne would eventually find a new career after her hiatus from working outside the home, that we would find a church for our family, and that our kids would attend good schools. Our old church in Cary was one of the things that was keeping us from contemplating moving in the first place; however, in the year leading up to our move to Greensboro and my accepting a position at UNC Greensboro, our church went through some internal struggles that made it easier for us move. We would miss the people of Greenwood Forest Baptist Church but not the conflict.

Something else keeping us in Cary was our success in getting into the magnet system of Wake County Public Schools via lottery. Lilli had gone to Fuller Elementary School, one of the Gifted and

Talented magnet elementary schools in the county, for kindergarten and first grade, and Amelia was registered to begin kindergarten in the fall of 2010. It took our leap of faith to leave that security of a great school and go to the unknown of Guilford County Schools. LouAnne had done her homework, though, and identified a few good neighborhood school districts with houses in our price range.

Lastly, it was our local Trader Joe's in Cary that was keeping us attached to Cary and the Triangle. While there was no Trader Joe's in Greensboro, we had faith that one would eventually move to a city like Greensboro that already had an Apple store. In late 2019, Trader Joe's is *finally* moving to Greensboro only a few miles from our house, and it only took nine years for us to get back to some of our favorite groceries without driving 30-45 minutes to Winston-Salem or Chapel Hill.

When we finally allowed ourselves to believe in the move from Cary to Greensboro, LouAnne and I started looking for churches. LouAnne grew up Southern Baptist, and I grew up United Methodist. As a married couple, we had attended an inter-denominational church in New Jersey and two Baptist churches in North Carolina. We were ready open to different denominations, including United Methodist Churches, given my background. My father's father's father was a Methodist preacher who preached at five country churches, including Philadelphia UMC in Putnam County, Georgia, where I grew up. We found Guilford College UMC in Greensboro in part because of its proximity to where we looked at houses but also because their preschool seemed similar to the one we were leaving in Cary. More importantly, their preschool director was the first person to respond to LouAnne's e-mails to register Collin for preschool that fall.

Collin grew up in the church's preschool. The girls grew up in the children's program at the church. LouAnne and I found a home in the New Growth Sunday school class, and all of us got involved in various ways with different ministries and programs. We grew as a family of five, spiritually and physically, and the people in our church became like family.

From the moment we found out that Lilli had a serious illness, our church family at Guilford College UMC was there for us. Lilli wasn't even in the church's youth group as a sixth grader, but the youth minister had been notified by someone the night that Lilli was in the emergency room. That youth minister contacted our senior pastor, who showed up at Lilli's door within hours of Lilli's being admitted. Our Sunday school class organized the Meal Train account, some of the initial meals for our family, and visited us almost daily in the hospital for the first few weeks.

We weren't about to abandon our church. It was hard, however, for me to go to Sunday school regularly, as I could only go on alternate Sundays. It was also difficult to sit in a small group, the primary structure of our class, and have an intimate discussion. Although I had gotten used to the question, "How is Lilli," and had a boiler plate answer to it, I couldn't engage folks in a deep conversation about what it's like to be the parent of a cancer patient. Instead of going to Sunday school, I attended the formal worship service during Lilli's treatments. Like most worship services I've attended since I was a young lad, our church allows folks to worship in a passive manner, which suited me. I could still attend church but could maintain some distance between myself and the other congregants. I tried not to make too much eye contact while worshipping, as I would've broken down in tears.

Our church helped organize many fundraisers for our family, too. Some of the classes and members from the church also donated money to help us out. There were times when people would come up to me without warning and hand me an envelope with a check or cash or a simple note of encouragement. The youth group raised money for our family through its biannual consignment sale. And several times there were anonymous donor guardian angels who helped us pay off our medical bills. We needed our church to get through our ordeal and not go bankrupt.

Round Two

While early on the team gave us the impression that Lilli would have a week between rounds of chemo, it wasn't as generous as that. After her first month of chemo one of her doctors said, "We don't want to give the cancer any chance to reestablish itself. As soon as her body's ready, we'll go back and attack the cancer as quickly as possible." We had only a few days between coming home from Lilli's first round and going back for the next one. The second round consisted of eight straight days of chemo, virtually around the clock, followed by three weeks of recovery. Lilli was back in room 912, our old familiar room, and I felt some comfort in knowing that she had previously done well in this room and that she had also escaped the room by going home once her counts came up.

At the beginning of round two we heard from Lilli's doctors how impressed they were that her body had responded well to the chemotherapy and that it appeared that her cancer was in remission.

What do they mean, "Her body responded so well?" Are they really just trying to say that the chemotherapy didn't kill her as much as it killed the cancer cells? Was it really her body that responded well or the cancer cells that responded poorly? I guess this phrase is just the way they'll talk about this, so I'll repeat it for anyone else who's familiar with cancer talk. "Oh, yes, she's responding so well to the chemo," I'll tell them when they ask.

The news that her body was responding well gave me hope that she would not need a bone marrow transplant and that the chemotherapy alone might do the job to kill all the cancer cells. Dr. Russell said that we would "keep the bone marrow transplant in our back pocket," just in case Lilli were to need one down the road. Dr. Russell mentioned that, even if there were no bone marrow match out there for Lilli, there were advances in using umbilical cord blood stem cells for bone marrow transplants and that there were definitely cord blood cells that would match Lilli's cells.

I felt more knowledgeable about the whole month-long process of Lilli's receiving three different chemotherapy drugs for the first week, a week or two of bottoming out of Lilli's blood counts, and a week of recovering. I had learned some of the drug names: Cytarabine, Daunorubicin, Etoposide, and I had even learned the trick of silencing the IV pole's beeping while we waited for a nurse. Even with that experience and knowledge, however, I was worried about the side effects of treatments. Lilli was starting to lose more of her hair, and I had to brace myself for the image of my precious girl's going bald. She didn't worry too much about losing her hair; instead, she spent time making golf-ball-sized hair balls and sculptures out of the hair that fell out. She rolled these balls around on the side of her bed and bedside table, and she added hair to them regularly. In addition to losing her hair, Lilli became lethargic and had a low appetite at the beginning of the second round.

Years earlier I would walk around campus at UNCG and think, "I wonder if Lilli will look like that student when she's in college. That student's mannerisms, build, clothes, and hair kind of remind me of Lilli's." Those thoughts were replaced with more fearful ones like, "I hope she lives long enough to go to college." I was trying to put hair into context by reminding myself that it should grow back at some point, but the time between a full head of hair and a bald head was hard to watch.

Once the isolation restrictions were lifted and the oncology team returned to their normal scrubs, the art and music therapists started showing up. With a long red beard and braids, Colin Allured, the music therapist, arrived with a cart full of musical instruments. He was a hippie-looking, easy going, loving guy with a flair for classical guitar, and he had a way with using music to touch Lilli and anyone else in the room. Colin would enter the room and ask calmly if Lilli wanted to work with him. Most times the answer was yes, but occasionally she would not feel up to it.

Colin taught Lilli a handful of basic chords on the baritone ukulele, an instrument that Lilli and I had ordered for LouAnne's Christmas present. The baritone uke stayed around Lilli's room so long that it became a loaner instrument for Lilli and one that she could keep in the room at all times. There is a video of Colin and

Lilli playing the 8-bar blues, Colin on guitar and Lilli on baritone uke, where Lilli is balancing a deck of playing cards on her head while playing the blues. Colin is that kind of musician with the ability to have fun with kids with the most life-threatening illnesses imaginable.

Lilli had played the violin since she was five years old, but she didn't want to touch it while she was in the hospital. Similarly, Lilli was an avid reader, devouring books at an incredible pace, before she was admitted to the hospital. While she was a patient in the hospital, however, she could not bear to read any of her books. She could read enough to work through her school work, but she didn't read any of the novels on her reading list or wish list.

Art therapists were more numerous and varied, as the hospital participated in the *Arts for Life* program. Some days Lilli would be up for working with the artists, mostly college student volunteers or paid interns, and other days Lilli was not well enough to focus on the art projects. A sweet young auburn-haired college student came in and asked if Lilli was in the mood to work on something. Lilli nodded her head after I pressed her on the issue, "Come on, LilliBug, it'll do you good to work on something." The art therapist gave Lilli a few choices of things that she could do, from paintings to drawings to other arts and crafts, and Lilli picked out an owl-themed painting to work on with the art therapist that day.

Another program offered through the 9th floor clinic child life team, sponsored by several nonprofits in the area, was the *Beads of Courage* program. As a pediatric cancer patient Lilli was entered into this program that provided small plastic and glass beads of different colors and designs to represent different treatments and milestones along the way of her treatment. For example, there were different beads for losing hair, getting chemo, having a transfusion, spending the night in the hospital (Lilli got a lot of those), and special beads for completing all chemo treatments. Starting with beads that spelled her name and a cord to hold the beads, Lilli began collecting beads. She tracked her beads on a spreadsheet that LouAnne kept up with, and when we would see Stacy from the child life team we would ask her to update Lilli's beads. I'm not sure how many strands of beads the average patient accumulates, but Lilli the AML patient was racking up beads at a rapid pace.

Lilli spiked a fever one night during her second round of chemo (for that fever, Lilli would get a new bead), and she started losing energy. Fevers were one of my biggest fears, and I kept praying that Lilli would not spike a fever, as they signified some kind of virus or bacterial infection that Lilli's body was fighting. And when her white blood counts were essentially zero, an infection could be the most life-threatening experience, even worse than the chemotherapy itself. As I learned more about patients who died while fighting cancer, I learned that not all those patients died from the cancer, per se. Some of the patients were dying from infections arising from compromised immune systems.

Lilli's fever sprang into motion the standard protocol of the nurse's drawing blood cultures that would be sent to the lab to see if anything would grow from Lilli's blood, potentially revealing a source of the infection causing the fevers. Virtually all of Lilli's cultures grew nothing; however, Lilli continued to get fevers off and on.

Later during that round, Lilli spiked a fever that lasted for five days. My Aunt Teresa was staying at our house for a week to give my in-laws a break to go home and take care of business, pay bills, and check on their house. That week back in Greensboro, Collin also got sick to his stomach, threw up, chugged a PowerAde, threw up a lot more, and eventually got better. In our pre-cancer world, such an event would've been cause for concern, but a little vomit and an upset stomach were mild compared to what Lilli was dealing with in the hospital. Aunt Teresa sprayed Lysol all over Collin's bedroom and bathroom. "Whenever we get sick at my house, I just spray Lysol all over the place," she said. With Collin's stomach weaker than his sisters', he needed to recover by starting with light toast and saltines. After Aunt Teresa made him some toast, Collin for months referred to her as "that lady who makes good toast."

Aunt Teresa rode with me to the hospital to visit Lilli one day when the pediatric infectious disease team stopped by. When they walked in the room, en masse, it reminded me of those hospital shows on TV that LouAnne watches. The lead doctor walked in first, and a group of interns and fellows followed a few steps behind him. This doctor was part genius, part stand-up comedian. He had a great rapport with Lilli and cracked a lot of jokes with us. He said that Lilli looked way too good for him to be there. He said that while the numbers were important and the results from cultures were, too, the doctors still balanced their assessments with how the patient looked overall. He said that Lilli was tough to figure out, because she had been feverish for days but still looked like a healthy cancer patient. "She's an enigma," he said.

I looked over at Aunt Teresa who was on the sofa by the window, and her eyes grew big. She happened to visit on a pretty exciting day in the life of Lilli the leukemia patient. The doctor continued, "Yeah, we don't always figure out what it is causing patients to become febrile. We can determine the cause only about 25% of the time. Most of the time we never find out, and the patient recovers from whatever was causing the fever."

How comforting…NOT! So…Lilli could have some unknown infection from some undetermined disease caused by God-knows-what…and they can't tell us what's going on?! What kind of expertise is this?

The doctor needed a brighter light to examine Lilli. He struggled with his iPhone flashlight, and one of the interns helped him figure out how to turn it on and off. He gave Lilli just a few tests, like using the old tongue depressor and asking her to "say ah," feeling her lymph nodes, and looking in her ears, eyes, and mouth. He said he was comfortable with the treatment plan of high-dose antibiotics and with the specific meds that were being administered. I felt a little more reassured after his visit, but I couldn't wait until the fever subsided.

With the exception of the unknown bug that caused a five-day-long fever, Lilli's second month-long round of chemo and recovery went well. She missed out on sibling love, but she was able to connect with her school via Skype and the amazing video they made to cheer her up. She maintained her weight during the second round by eating soups, burgers, chicken nuggets, popcorn, jelly beans, and pizza. For Valentine's Day, we investigated what it would take to print custom heart candies with #LilliSTRONG printed on them, and after some research we ordered enough candy for all the kids at Lilli's school to get a small pack of candy message hearts. Working on a project like these hearts took Lilli's mind off the fact that her brother and sister couldn't visit due to the flu restrictions, and it was a fun and tasty distraction.

Lilli stayed in good spirits although she suffered the extended fever and couldn't see her siblings or friends. During the second round, Lilli also saw less of her classmates because of the flu ban, but also because they had all gone back to school after the holidays.

It's hard to maintain interest in a hospital patient long-term when that patient's not in the immediate family. I can't blame Lilli's friends and acquaintances if they're not fully invested in her struggle. It's pretty easy to change the channel and get on with life. For this reason, I'm even more thankful for Lilli's friends who are sticking with her through multiple months of treatments.

When her counts bottomed out and Lilli received nearly daily blood or platelet transfusions, I didn't freak out. I had seen this during her first round, and I recognized this new normal for Lilli with these life-saving transfusions. With low hemoglobin counts, Lilli would become sluggish. LouAnne and I became quite perceptive in this regard and could tell when Lilli's hemoglobin dropped below her threshold. For one thing, we learned the nurses' trick of pressing Lilli's fingernails to check for blood flow. When Lilli's platelets were low, the signs were easier to identify. She could get a bloody nose, but more often her low platelet count presented as petechiae [pi-tee-kee-aye], small red dots that would appear like a rash on her skin. LouAnne and I looked out for these signs and were not shy about asking for transfusions when Lilli's counts were borderline.

It didn't take long after her counts bottomed out and Lilli got through the fever that her counts started to pick up. This time I knew to watch closely for the White Blood Count and Absolute Neutrophil Count. LouAnne and I would ask each morning for an update on the counts, and it wasn't long before we were able to take Lilli back home for a break between the second and third rounds of chemo.

Two rounds…we've survived HALF of the treatments that're planned for Lilli. She's still alive, and she gets to sleep in her own bed at least one more time. Thank you, God!

Finances

We had not yet gotten a bill from the hospital, but I sensed that it was just a matter of time before we'd be up to our ears in hospital bills. I didn't want to call the insurance company, as I dread talking to anyone from an insurance company, but I looked at some of the information about my work-related insurance policy. I figured we'd hit the maximum out-of-pocket section of our family policy that was connected to my state university's employee-plus-family policy. The university provided my insurance premiums as an employee benefit, but I had to pay extra for the family coverage with pre-tax dollars from my salary. With LouAnne's working part-time as a preschool music teacher and the 20% pay cut that I took to go from practice to teaching full-time, we could only afford the cheaper, 70%-30% plan which carried with it higher deductibles and higher out-of-pocket expenses. I had been lucky enough to check the cancer coverage boxes for each of our family members when I first started teaching at UNCG. I can't explain why I did, as most financial planners, I believe, would advise clients not to sign up for those extra layers of insurance. Whatever the benefits and costs, however, we would hit the family maximum after just a few days of Lilli's chemotherapy treatments in 2014 and hit it again after a few days into 2015. I knew that we would need help to be able to pay our bills once they started flowing in 2015.

We had already gotten help from our Sunday school class, and LouAnne came home one day from picking up Amelia and Collin from school with an envelope full of money from Lilli's old elementary school. On the outside was written "Once a Gator, Always a Gator," and inside was a wad of cash. Lilli's middle school had also collected an envelope full of money that the counselor Ms. Denny delivered to our hospital room one day after school. People from our church also wanted to donate to help us pay our bills and to have spending money for gas and food as we travelled back and forth to the hospital.

After giving it some thought, LouAnne and I decided to forego any online fundraisers, right or wrong, and instead to set up a savings account at our credit union and to share the account information with anyone who asked. We had faith that God would provide enough friends, family, and perfect strangers who would be willing to donate to our account and help us avoid bankruptcy. I called the credit union to ask what we'd have to do to set up this account and was advised to go to my nearest branch. One cold, rainy, grey morning between Christmas 2014 and New Year's, I drove to the credit union branch not too far from our house and asked to speak to someone there who could help me. I sat down with a lovely middle-aged woman with curly blonde hair in a navy pant suit, and I explained why I was setting up a new money market account. "My daughter was diagnosed with leukemia a few weeks ago, and we'd like to have an account where people can donate money to help us," I said.

"Oh, I'm sorry that you're going through this," she replied, and proceeded to help me set up the account. We both avoided eye contact for the remainder of that meeting, as either one or both of us might've broken down emotionally.

Within a few weeks, folks had deposited hundreds of dollars in our account, and every week or so we would check the account to find that someone had anonymously deposited some money into our account. Occasionally those donors would let us know who they were and how much they had donated, but there were some donors who remain anonymous to this day.

We asked the social worker from the pediatric oncology unit to help us know our options for seeking financial help from non-profits or from the hospital. She pointed out that there was financial support from the hospital's financial aid office on the ground floor of the older part of the hospital, and she told me where to find more information. One afternoon when Lilli was doing well in her room, I decided that I could afford to walk down to the main hospital level to the financial aid office. I walked into a dark, internal office suite with no windows to the outside world and waited in the reception line. I checked in and sat down to wait for the next financial counselor.

I had collected a few bits of financial information for this initial meeting, but I didn't have all the pieces necessary to complete the application. I met with a sweet, patient staffer who was very encouraging and supportive. She listened to my story about Lilli and about how we were living in the hospital for a month at a time. She asked me a few questions about our family's resources. Did we have jobs? Did we have retirement accounts? Did we have insurance? What kind of insurance did we have? Did we rent or own our home? Did we have any other assets? Did we have savings accounts? After she asked for some of this basic information, she made sure that I had all the application materials and knew what documents I'd have to bring back with me.

After that meeting, I scoured our house back in Greensboro for all the paperwork that I could find: our latest credit union statements, paystubs, insurance account numbers, and the like. I filled out the application, and I felt encouraged by some of the marketing materials from the financial aid office, suggesting that patient bills could be reduced significantly, even reduced to zero, depending on the patient's ability to pay the bills. Knowing that we would be up against tens of thousands of dollars in hospital bills, I was certain that we'd get some kind of support from the hospital. I was confident in our application's potential when I took all the information and paperwork back to the same person with whom I met the first time. She was just as sweet and encouraging, and she looked through the materials, made copies of the paperwork, returned the originals, and told me that we'd hear from the office in a few weeks after they had reviewed our application.

A few weeks later, I opened the mailbox to find a formal letter from the financial aid office.

They offered no reduction.

They offered nothing.

No discount.

No, nothing.

What? What's working against us? Can't they see we're already in debt from this back-and-forth hospital lifestyle? Do they really want us to drain our savings? Do they really want us to cash out our retirement accounts? Do they really want us to sell everything we own? Take out a second mortgage? I guess we get no help because we still have jobs, insurance, and retirement accounts. Will they help us only once we're bankrupt? I wouldn't want any patient to go without treatment, but we'd almost be better off if we were completely destitute.

If we had been wealthy, then we'd have had no trouble paying. If we had been destitute, then they'd zero out our bill. We were too rich to get help and too poor to pay. Even with all the help we got from friends, family, strangers, our church, co-workers, neighbors, and others, we'd be affected for years to come, both physically and fiscally.

Round Three

Lilli returned to Brenner for the third of four month-long rounds of chemo. Like the previous two months, Lilli had a bone marrow aspirate. While the team had her knocked out for that, they did a spinal tap to check for signs of cancer in her spinal fluid and also injected some chemo into her spinal fluid. When the team shared the results with us later that day, we heard the same good news that we heard with the previous rounds: no signs of cancer in her spinal fluid.

Whew! I'm glad that there are no signs of cancer in her spinal fluid. Leukemia that goes to the brain through the spine scares me, and I'm thankful that we haven't had to deal with that level of cancer.

Lilli was taken back to room 912, our old familiar pressurized room, and she got a bite to eat after having to fast overnight for that morning's procedures. Later that afternoon, Lilli started getting the chemotherapy that was planned for round three: five straight days of chemo, this time only two of the three main drugs that she had received the first two rounds. Lilli was happy not to have to take the one that made her sicker than the others. With the chemo came the nurses in hazmat suits. They warned us not to come in contact with the chemicals and not to touch Lilli's sweat or other bodily fluids during the days she was getting chemo. With each round, the number of days decreased, from ten days in round one to eight days in round two and now five days for round three.

Each chemo drug was infused via IV into Lilli's central line. If I had sat down to dwell on the drugs, I would've lost sleep over the toxic chemicals being pumped into Lilli's body; instead, I pretended like these chemo infusions were normal, like walking and talking. One of the drugs was neon pink, like something out of science fiction, and it turned Lilli's urine bright pink, too. There was a limit to the amount of toxins that Lilli's body could handle, and the AML roadmap nearly accounted for the lifetime toxicity limits on our baby girl's body.

After the doctors had a chance to look at the bone marrow sample under the microscope, they told us that they liked what they saw. They said that it still looked like Lilli's cancer was in remission, and they felt good about continuing on the roadmap as planned. At each turn, it seemed like things were too good to be true. After being told that Lilli had leukemia, I had prepared myself mentally for the worst. However, with each subsequent test, lab result, and Lilli's body's response to the chemo, Lilli seemed to be the model AML patient.

After receiving the chemo, Lilli's blood counts dropped like a rock about a week later. While the notion of keeping track of blood counts was foreign to me the first month, I had become a hawk about tracking Lilli's counts. Although other counts would be tracked, we focused on the three primary markers on a daily basis once Lilli's body neared the bottom of each month. 1) WBC: White Blood Count, which would go to zero by the time Lilli bottomed out (white blood cells fight against infections). 2) HGB: Hemoglobin, a measure of red blood that, without persistent blood transfusions, would also be zero at the bottom (red blood circulates oxygen through the bloodstream). And 3) PLT: Platelets, which also required vigilance and multiple transfusions (platelets cause blood to clot to keep it from thinning). For days Lilli's White Blood Count remained at zero. During those days Lilli couldn't go out of the room and had to be careful about having guests. With no defense against infections, Lilli had to trust each visitor with her life. I tried not to become paranoid about visitors, but I kept watch for signs of any illnesses like runny eyes, sniffling, and sneezing.

Lilli was a model patient, but she couldn't avoid some of the side effects of the chemo and the resulting depletion of her immune system. About halfway through the third round, Lilli developed a skin rash that her team inspected very carefully. After consulting with each other, the team came back with a recommendation to take Lilli off the chlorhexidine wipes study, the only medical trial that we agreed to do. Lilli wasn't upset in the least to be able to stop wiping herself down with these wipes every day, and I was relieved that the skin rash was nothing more serious. Lilli also developed a cough and congestion during this round, which reminded me of the cough she had the week before she was diagnosed in 2014. Lilli also spiked a few fevers during round three, triggering IV antibiotics from her friend *Beepy* the IV pole, but the fevers subsided quickly, each within 12 hours. While each of these side effects kept me on my toes with anxiety, the third round of chemo could've been a lot worse for all of us.

Lilli made the most of being in the hospital for the third month in a row. The hospital's lifting the flu restrictions on young visitors that month meant that Lilli could have sleepovers, and her sister and brother took turns spending the night at the hospital for two weekends in a row in March. As the weather improved, LouAnne took the kids to the rooftop playground for the first time. They were able to play together and take in the beautiful skyline view of Winston-Salem. Lilli enjoyed doing more arts and crafts with the Arts-for-Life team, and she learned a few more tunes on the baritone ukulele from Colin, the music therapist. Lilli took ownership over her room décor, and she added some string lights, accessories, and some of her own artwork to the walls and the wall-to-wall windowsill. With the help of her appetite stimulant medication, Lilli maintained her weight by eating popcorn, cheeseburgers, and jelly beans and by drinking V-8, apple juice, and Starbucks hot chocolate. No other hot chocolate appealed to her.

As Lilli's blood counts started to increase, we got word from the Make-A-Wish staff that Lilli's application for a wish was approved. A team of two staffers from Make-A-Wish stopped by Lilli's room one evening to interview our family and talk to Lilli about her wish. Lilli had already dreamed about the family trip she envisioned from her wish. Lilli studied some of the local attractions in Navarre, FL, on her tablet, and I had emailed the staff Lilli's top ten list. They came to the hospital one evening bearing a small bag of gifts and hope for our family that we would be able to take a trip together in spite of Lilli's fight against leukemia.

One morning the nurse came in to check on Lilli, and I asked if Lilli's counts were back from the blood drawn the night before. The nurse checked and let us know that Lilli's ANC had jumped from 0 to 100. The team liked for the ANC to be moving at or close to 500 before discharging Lilli, and it seemed like Lilli would be going home sooner than anticipated. The following morning, LouAnne got the counts from the team. Lilli's ANC had dropped back down to zero. Discouraged by the up and down counts, we asked the team what it meant. "Oh, this is fairly standard for patients. There's often some up and down of counts as the bone marrow recovers," Dr. McLean assured us. I couldn't help but be concerned by this jumping around of Lilli's counts, no matter what the team did or said to reassure us.

While LouAnne and I continued to swap off at the hospital, maintain our careers, and maintain some semblance of home with the help of our family, our community continued to come together to help us out. There was great turnout for a pizza fundraiser at the Greensboro Brixx restaurant. My sister, Tammy, came to town for a week to give my in-laws a break, and she stayed at the hospital with Lilli the evening of the pizza fundraiser. This allowed me and LouAnne to go together with Amelia and Collin for some pizza on a cold and wet evening. We saw many of our friends from church, schools, and our community, and they collectively bought and ate over 300 pizzas to raise money for our family. My faith in humanity was renewed over and over again during Lilli's treatments, and that evening at BRIXX was one source of that renewal.

Once Lilli's ANC rebounded for good, the team discharged her. We had a streamlined storage and packing system by that point, after two previous months of chemo, and it took less time for us to roll our storage bins down to the parking deck and leave Winston-Salem in our rearview mirror. "One more round, and we're done," I thought. I was optimistic and scared to death.

What if this final round doesn't do the trick? What if the cancer comes back? I have to trust the process and the expertise of Lilli's oncology team and try to maintain my faith and trust in God to lead us.

Round Four

After three rounds of chemo that had the same kind of rhythm, 5-10 days of chemo followed by three weeks of recovery, round four was a totally different chemo cocktail. Lilli would have only one chemo drug via IV infusion followed by a new drug administered by needle injections. Her bone marrow aspirate still showed signs of remission, and the spinal tap still showed no cancer cells going to her brain. Lilli was a pro at all these procedures that scared the dickens out of me.

After just two days of being inpatient, Lilli was discharged from the hospital to spend a few days at home. The new regimen threw us off our stride, but I wasn't complaining about having more of my LilliBug at home. LouAnne was with Lilli when the team administered her final chemo via injections. She called me so that I could be part of the ceremonial end of Lilli's chemotherapy. The nurses counted down, and LouAnne held the phone where I could hear their excitement. The doctor that weekend gave Lilli the chemo injections, first one thigh, then the other. There was cheering, applause, and a few tears when we celebrated the end to Lilli's treatments.

Dr. McLean, the head of pediatric oncology who was on the unit's schedule that week, gave Lilli a four-day pass to leave the hospital and spend some time at home before coming back for the low period of Lilli's blood counts. Having Lilli at home with Amelia and Collin gave me a glimpse of what it would be like to have all three kids at home together again. The kids had fun playing video games together, playing with the neighbors, and fussing and fighting like typical siblings.

I had to temper my enthusiasm with the reminder that Lilli wasn't completely done and that we'd have to keep her safe through yet another depletion of her immune system, which she would do once she was readmitted to the oncology unit. LouAnne drove Lilli back to the hospital on a day when I had to teach, and she called me from the hospital to let me know that Lilli had NOT, in fact, completed all the chemo.

What?! Why was there any ceremony around the shots you gave her last week? Don't they know what they're doing?

"The nurses weren't quite sure what was going on, either," LouAnne said. "It's been a few years since they've had an AML patient here, and some of the nurses weren't here back then."

LouAnne told me that the fourth month was actually designed to administer the chemo in two halves with a few days in between, so Lilli returned to the hospital with some unfinished work. She'd have to go through the infusions of one chemo followed by the same ceremonial injections of chemo in her thighs. Once again, LouAnne was the parent on duty the day when Lilli had those injections, and LouAnne had me on speaker phone again when the doctor injected Lilli with her final doses of chemo. This time we asked the team to tell us if this was, once and for all, the end of Lilli's treatments. For real? For real, for real? And it was.

After those final injections, we had another familiar period of wait-and-see as Lilli's bone marrow was depleted and had to rebuild itself. The doctors warned us that, due to the differences in the fourth round of chemo, it could take up to five or six weeks for Lilli's counts to recover. We were familiar with the three-week rhythm, but I braced myself for a longer, more drawn out recovery during which Lilli would require a lot of blood and platelet transfusions.

In the midst of all these treatments, our community hosted more fundraisers. Lilli was getting some of her final chemo infusions and injections as McAllister's Deli hosted a fundraiser for our family. While LouAnne was in the hospital with Lilli, I was able to attend the fundraiser with Amelia, Collin, Joe, and Janet. McAllister's was one of several restaurants, including Brixx Pizza, that helped our family with medical bills.

We encouraged Lilli's classmates to come to the hospital to visit Lilli on days when she felt well. Most of her classmates who visited came with their moms, and several of the moms asked how Lilli was able to keep up with homework. To be honest, Lilli had lost some steam in completing her schoolwork, especially since the Winston-Salem Forsyth County school system was on Spring

Break. Lilli's hospital teacher Jamie wasn't at the hospital for a week, and the following week Lilli's home school would be on break. I made a request for some homework buddies to visit after school to work on problems, mostly math, with Lilli so that she could not only keep up with her homework but also hang out with her friends. A few of Lilli's friends came to the hospital with their moms, and they worked on math before socializing like normal sixth graders.

Around the middle of Lilli's fourth month of chemo, my sister Tammy came to visit for a week to give Joe and Janet a chance to check on their home. Tammy was able to help LouAnne work on our house to prepare it for Lilli to come home for good. During Spring Break, Amelia and Collin were able to spend more time with their sister who hosted a handful of sleepovers at the hospital. The siblings by this time were no strangers to all the doctors and nurses who encouraged as much quality time as possible between all three of our kids. They recognized how Lilli's mood was improved by having her brother and sister around the hospital.

Lilli's friends from Greensboro were also out on break, so we had a flood of young pre-teen girls visiting the room. They spent some time playing on the rooftop playground and enjoyed seeing a part of Winston that they would've never seen without having a friend in the hospital. One day a group of these girls stopped by when Colin, the music therapist, was there. Being the great person he is, Colin broke out all kinds of instruments for all the people in the room. Lilli had the baritone ukulele that she'd been learning from Colin, and the other girls got various drums, keyboards, and other rhythm instruments. Lilli's spirits were lifted by Colin's leading them all through a concert of *Let it Go* from Frozen and Katy Perry's *Firework*.

Lilli was having a great week. The visitors cheered her up. She enjoyed hanging out with her brother and sister. They spent some time at the rooftop playground, too, and I loved watching my three kids spend time together. After nearly four months we had learned to make a home away from home out of our hospital room. I got to know most of the staff in the pediatric hematology-oncology unit, and I was comfortable with the whole experience. Lilli looked stronger and healthier than she had since November before her diagnosis. I was starting to look forward to a time when Lilli would be totally finished with the hospital life and would be able to return home for good.

And just when I thought we were in the clear, Lilli spiked a fever one night during the low period of this round of chemo. She had required a few blood and platelet transfusions already during this round, but she hadn't spiked a fever since the previous round. Overnight, Lilli lost the freedom she had from *Beepy* and had to be reconnected to the pole with an IV antibiotic. The fever subsided on its own by the following morning, but none of us could've foreseen what was about to happen. Cancer and its side effects were about to scare the life out of me.

PICU

....

"Most AML patients spend time in the PICU with each round. Y'all are lucky that this was your first time."

Those words from one of our favorite nurses came as little comfort to me as I had just experienced the closest Lilli had ever come to death.

The day before had started out like normal. Lilli felt well that morning. She was in bed catching up on arts and crafts and HGTV. I asked what she wanted for lunch. That day it was Chick-fil-A, a short drive down the road. When Lilli was feeling well, I wouldn't think twice about driving out for lunch, leaving her alone for a brief while, and that day she was perfectly fine to stay by herself. After I came back with lunch for the two of us I could tell that Lilli wasn't herself. While she ate some of the lunch, she had lost her appetite and couldn't finish it. She told me, "I'm tired, Daddy. I just want to rest." She rolled over and pulled the blanket over her and slid the eye mask over her eyes. Lilli had a collection of eye masks that she used religiously in the hospital because of all the lights and lack of privacy when she needed to rest. She curled up under all the covers.

I had spent enough time with Lilli in the hospital that I was pretty good at just looking at her and being able to tell whether or not she had a fever without a thermometer. I watched her breathing intensify and become heavier and more labored. I felt Lilli's arm and forehead, and she was burning up. Her temperature was going up, up, and up. I pressed Lilli's bedside call button and called on the nurse to come in and check her temperature. By that time, it was over 100.4, which meant an automatic blood draw for cultures to figure out the cause of the fever, if possible. Following that draw, the nurse went back out to the station and to attend to other patients. Lilli's body continued to heave more rapidly, more than normal as it got hotter, and I called on the nurse again to come back and check on Lilli. Her temperature was over 102 and rising. This was the fastest I had ever seen her body temp rise, and I started to worry. I texted LouAnne, who was on her way, "Get here as quickly as possible!!!! Lilli's got a fever, and it's HIGH." LouAnne was driving and didn't answer her texts. I texted over and over again, about every five minutes.

"Where are you?"

"LouAnne?"

"LouAnne?!!!"

I texted Tammy, too, who was supposed to be riding with LouAnne that afternoon. We had hatched a plan, because Lilli had been doing so well, for Amelia and Collin to spend the night with Lilli and have a family sleepover while Tammy drove back home to look after our house. There was no response from Tammy, either.

Lilli's fever was a little above 105 before the rest of the family got there. By that time all the nurses and doctors on the unit were alerted to what was going with Lilli. One of the *twin* nurses (really two unrelated nurses who, to me, looked like twins, and I couldn't tell them apart except for one worked nights and the other worked days) took Lilli's temperature with Dr. Russell in the room, and it was 105.6. I repeat: 105.6! When the nurse saw the thermometer, she turned quickly towards me and Dr. Russell with a look of shock and dismay in her eyes that told me "This is serious!"

I still hadn't heard a response to my texts when I saw LouAnne, Tammy, Collin, and Amelia arrive through the vestibule window. As soon as they walked into the vestibule, though, Lilli vomited in their direction, all over the floor between her bed and the bathroom. She had given me a little warning, saying that her stomach didn't feel well. I did my best to grab a pan and catch as much as I could, but it was all over the place, and I was straddling it as best I could. LouAnne and Tammy said that they hadn't checked their texts while they were on the road and that they were trying to get to the room quickly. They didn't stop to check texts on the way up to the 9th floor from the parking deck, either. It was news to them that Lilli was feverish, and the shock hit them as soon as they saw the anguish on my face. We asked Tammy to take Collin and Amelia to the rooftop playground so they could get out of the way and not see their big sister so sick. LouAnne and I turned our undivided attention to Lilli.

Before long the nursing team, led by one of the senior nurses, Jo, whom we mostly saw on weekends and nights, brought in a large bag of cold fluids to push into Lilli's system to try to cool her body temperature. I had never seen the team move this quickly. There was a flurry of activity with nurses coming in and out. While I was inwardly concerned for Lilli, I didn't know exactly how concerned to be, as I had not seen anything like this. Jo began to extract fluids with a huge syringe from the bags and push them directly into Lilli's central line, another sight I had not seen. The IV drip just wouldn't allow the cold fluids to be pushed quickly enough, Jo said, so she used this big syringe to do the job.

At that same time, they hooked up Lilli to all the gauges and monitors, keeping tabs on her heart rate, blood pressure, and oxygen levels, among other things. Her breathing became heavy. Her heart rate skyrocketed. Her blood pressure plummeted. I had gotten used to most of the bells, dings, and pings from *Beepy*, and I could tell the difference between normal and not-normal sounds. Lilli had become a veritable sound and light show of not-normal that afternoon. Her blood pressure had dropped to a dangerously low level. The team attempted to stabilize her through the fluids and I suspect a few other things that I missed in all the action of folks running in and out of the room.

One of Lilli's friends was supposed to come over that evening to hang out with Amelia and Lilli for some arts and crafts. LouAnne texted her mom to let her know what was going on and not to come to the hospital. Instead, LouAnne asked the mom to start a prayer chain of folks praying for Lilli's health throughout the night. I doubled down on that request with a quick Facebook post, asking folks to "pray real hard."

Dr. Russell came back in after an hour or so of this hive of activity around Lilli. I stood five feet away from Lilli's bed the entire time, frozen. I couldn't move towards Lilli and get in the way of the team, but I couldn't force myself to lose focus on her during that time, either. Dr. Russell said, "I think that the scary part has passed." By that time, Lilli's temperature had gone down, closer to 100.

Wait! That was scary to you?! You mean you don't see this every day? You're an oncologist who has witnessed all kinds of things. For you to be scared means I should be scared TO DEATH. You all hid your fears from me by being so calm and professional as you cared for Lilli. Please God, let Lilli live through this.

I still don't know how scared they were for Lilli's life, and I probably never will. The scary part had passed, but by that time it was time for the daytime oncology team to turn over the patients to the nighttime guard of interns and fellows who would look after Lilli through the night after the 7:00pm shift change. Dr. Russell explained that he had given the night team instructions to transfer Lilli to the Pediatric Intensive Care Unit, or PICU, if she didn't show signs of improvement. He explained that he had also called down to the PICU to make sure they were aware of Lilli's case and prepared for her transfer, if that were how it would turn out.

"Do you feel better now that you've thrown up, Lilli?" Dr. Russell asked.

"Yeah, a little bit," Lilli replied.

We told the team that we had planned on having a sleepover that night and that Lilli's brother and sister had come to visit and stay the night. We all agreed that there might be an emotional benefit to having Amelia spend the night and have some sister bonding time but to have Collin go back home with Aunt Tammy and come back in a day or two when Lilli was feeling better. Before Tammy left, I said a prayer that God would look after and Lilli and that he would help her through the night.

After all of this we still had to figure out what to do about dinner. Not that any of us had any appetite for dinner, but we had learned to look after ourselves enough to have the energy to take care of Lilli when needed. I ran out and across the street to Cagney's Diner for boxed dinners for all of us. Each time I left Lilli in a situation where she wasn't 100%, I couldn't keep my mind off her and the possibility that she could get worse when I wasn't there. The manager of the diner, with whom I had spoken a few times about Lilli, asked how she was doing. I couldn't respond. My face burned with emotion. He put his hand on my shoulder and said that he'd be praying for her. When I returned to the hospital room carrying our dinners, including a few surprise desserts compliments of the manager, Lilli and Amelia were in bed together doing some online shopping, another favorite pastime of our cancer patient. There seemed to be a bit of healing just from Lilli's being with her sister.

I couldn't erase the experience earlier that day from my mind, though, and I asked the nurses for a thermometer that we could keep in the room. I drove Lilli and LouAnne crazy, checking Lilli's temperature every 10-15 minutes, as I worried that she might spike another fever. Most nights I would hold my breath while my heart rate spiked at the thought of Lilli's temperature check. I dreaded vitals checks. The CNAs, or Certified Nursing Assistants, would check her temperature periodically, about every four hours, when they also checked her blood pressure and oxygen. I would pray that there would be no fever and that her vitals would be normal, but I would also fear the worst whenever they would show up to check her vitals. I had a love-hate relationship with the thermometer. On one hand, I never wanted to know the results of the temperature check. On the other hand, I wanted the team to treat Lilli for any virus or bacterial infection that caused an elevated temp. That night I kept checking Lilli's temperature and pacing back and forth worrying about all the bells and whistles going off on the IV pole monitors. We heard a lot from our friend *Beepy* that night.

As we all prepared to go to sleep for the night, the team of interns and fellows came in periodically to check on Lilli. The nurses and CNAs did the same, more frequently than normal. The lead doctor on the night team kept commenting on how Lilli looked better clinically than she did on the monitors. "She's a puzzle," she said to us. "She shouldn't look as good as she does." I kept praying to myself that Lilli would improve inside and out and not need a transfer down to the PICU. I had heard stories of other kids' being admitted to the PICU and staying there for weeks or months before being transferred back to a normal patient room. I had also imagined that the PICU would be only one step away from death and wished that Lilli would never have to go down there.

In the middle of the night Lilli's blood pressure had barely increased. Her body was still in shock from whatever hit her so hard earlier in the day. The team leader, a strong young female doctor with her hair pulled back and wearing loose grey scrubs, decided that it was time to transfer Lilli to the PICU where she would be watched more closely. This was not the way I envisioned the night going, but it was clear that the team was seriously concerned about Lilli's health. LouAnne and I agreed that I would be the one to escort Lilli down to the PICU and that LouAnne would stay with Amelia who was asleep on our Kisses4Kate sleeping pad on the floor. I was stunned to watch Lilli and her bed being wheeled out of the room, in reverse from when she was initially wheeled up to the 9th floor back in December. One of Lilli's favorite nurses Mary was the one to walk us down to the PICU and into the glass fishbowl of a room where Lilli would be monitored.

Despite the glass storefront facing a long nurses' station and staff work area, the room was cold and dark compared to Lilli's old 9th floor room. There were no pictures all over the wall, no get-well cards, no arts and crafts. If the 9th floor room had a lot of life-saving gadgets on the wall, it paled in comparison to this PICU room. The whole room was laid out for life-saving efficiency. There were devices I had never seen before mounted on the ceiling above the bed and on every wall surface in sight, except for a small sofa tucked into the exterior wall near a small window with a view to the exterior wall of another building in the large hospital complex. What an austere, institutional, clinical, sterile environment to try to recover and regain one's life! I couldn't bear to think about losing Lilli in a space like this. There wasn't much about the space that encouraged recovery.

I texted LouAnne as soon as we got settled into the PICU room that we had made it. I stood for a long time with my eyes fixed on the readout from all the nodes and lines attached to Lilli. Her blood pressure slowly increased as soon as we got down there. LouAnne texted back that Mary mentioned the concept of a therapeutic transfer and that we'd be blessed if Lilli could experience such a thing. Lilli was not only fighting to recover from whatever attacked her the day before but also trying to rebuild her bone marrow's production of blood cells. She was at the bottom of her fourth month in this four-month road map, and she still needed regular blood transfusions.

The PICU nurse, a stranger to us, was a far cry from the 9th floor nurses who had become like family members to us. Lilli knew all her old nurses by name and by their likes and dislikes. This PICU nurse? She had a long way to go before she gained that same level of familiarity with Lilli, and Lilli couldn't wait to get back to her team of doctors and nurses upstairs. By the time Dr. Russell rounded that morning, Lilli's blood pressure was still going up and was almost back to the low end of a normal range. Dr. Russell suggested that if Lilli's body could continue to recover at this pace, then she might be able to go back upstairs the next day. He said that the team wanted to keep her in the PICU for observation for at least 24 hours.

This plan did not suit Lilli at all. All day long she kept talking about how much she missed her old room.

Imagine that...a 12-year-old girl wishing to be in a pediatric cancer room. We've gotten to that point, where there's something worse to our daughter than being stuck in a hospital room. It's being stuck in a fishbowl of an intensive care unit.

I left the PICU unit briefly that day when LouAnne came to see Lilli and to sit with her for a while. Amelia was in Lilli's old room upstairs with Tammy and Collin, and I went back up there to take a shower and to check on Amelia. That day we would all take turns watching different kids in different places, taking advantage of the Ronald McDonald House's family support room on the same floor as the PICU, and swapping off in Lilli's fishbowl. Walking into Lilli's old 9th floor room with no bed took my breath away. The room was there, but my baby girl wasn't where she was supposed to be. I had a glimpse of the worst possibility imaginable.

My daughter isn't guaranteed to make it back here. Is this the way it goes for kids who never make it out of PICU? Will they let us keep this room overnight? Will they kick us out?

I walked out to the nurses' station and asked them if we could keep Lilli's room for at least one more night, as it looked like there was a good chance she could be back the following day. They agreed to keep our room for another day, waiting for Lilli to return, but that they'd have to give it to someone else if Lilli were to stay in the PICU for longer. While I was talking to the 9th floor team, Jamie stopped by to see what was up. He had heard that Lilli was in the PICU and said he'd be praying for her and the rest of us. The whole team had heard what was going on and told us they were praying for us. And then one of Lilli's favorite nurses told us about most AML patients' needing to stay in the PICU at least once every month of their chemo treatments. We were the lucky ones to have made it through 3.5 months of treatment without a visit to the PICU.

141

People tried to comfort me, and I tried to repeat their words to myself: *At least Lilli is in a place where she'll get the most attention and constant care in the hospital. But wait! Shouldn't every space in a hospital provide that same level of care? I know better than to believe that lie, though.*

After I showered, changed clothes, and returned to the PICU, I asked Dr. Russell for his plans. He was still set on leaving Lilli in the PICU overnight. Though it took a lot to upset Lilli, this plan really upset her, to the point where I could tell she was getting choked up. After Dr. Russell left the room, LouAnne and I talked to Lilli about this plan. Her blood pressure was back in the normal range by mid-afternoon, and the blood for her transfusion was on its way. When Dr. Russell came back to check in one last time, we begged him to let Lilli go back upstairs to her room, as long as he was comfortable with her recovery. He talked very seriously to Lilli and asked about her emotional and mental state of mind. He was supportive, taking into account Lilli's maturity and how her body had recovered, of letting her go back upstairs and of keeping a close eye on her, with PICU at the ready in case she had to return.

Just what was it that Lilli had fought off, with the quick action and attentive care of the 9th floor team? We later were told that it was most likely sepsis, a blood infection, and septic shock that made her vital organs go haywire and, if not for the actions of the team that day, could've killed her.

Sepsis?! That's what ultimately killed Mohammed Ali, isn't it?! Lilli could've died right there and then, but she was spared this time.

How great to see Lilli back in her 9th floor hospital room that evening, even though I was nervous about her blood pressure and temperature. She was munching on Doritos and watching Netflix, like nothing had happened. She had survived, however, the most difficult 36 hours of her four months. I tried to make light of our ordeal by telling Lilli and the nurses that the leukemia just wouldn't let us leave the hospital without at least one visit to the PICU and that the leukemia had its last gasp before being totally beaten by Lilli and the chemo.

By the weekend Lilli was more or less back to her old self. The nurses finally removed the vital sign monitors and leads from her body, giving her a bit more freedom to move around the room. The friend who was supposed to come and do some arts and crafts with her the night of her infection came to visit. The two of them hung out in the room, coloring, cutting, and pasting various craft projects while Amelia and Collin visited. Collin had discovered the video game carts on the unit, and he put in a request for the next available cart.

"We need to make sure all the patients have had a turn with the video games before you play, son," I said. He understood, but that didn't keep him from asking about the carts every 5-10 minutes. His CNA buddy Marcia could sense that his whispering meant something, and she asked what it was he was talking about. And then she walked us down to the closet where they kept the video game carts, bins full of hats for the patients, shelves full of quilts, blankets, and pillows (like the ones in Lilli's room her first night), and the scales to weigh patients. Collin picked out the cart with one of his favorite video games, and we rolled it back to Lilli's room where Collin disappeared into his own gaming world for several hours.

LouAnne mentioned that friends had been asking when Lilli would get to ring the bell. Ring what bell?? I hadn't seen any bell. I had to look online to see what she was talking about. Apparently, cancer patients have a tradition of ringing a ceremonial bell, usually hanging in a clinic area, at the end of their treatments. Lilli had already gotten her final chemo shots a few weeks earlier, but with AML she had spent almost all of her time inpatient and not in the clinic. While other patients spent most of their hospital visits in the clinic, Lilli's experience was the opposite. We hadn't even gotten to know the clinic staff. I made a mental note to look for a bell and to ask about it once Lilli was definitely finished with her treatments and when cancer was in our rearview mirror.

Going Home

The team was correct when they said that Lilli's bone marrow recovery would probably be a little slower. Her neutrophils remained at 0% to 1% for nearly a week. The white blood counts and neutrophil counts inched up, ever so slowly, but Lilli couldn't shake a low-grade fever. After what happened the previous week with our sepsis run-in, the oncology team wasn't going to take any chances. Lilli was able to go 12 hours, 24 hours, and even 36 hours without a fever, but low-grade fevers in the 101 to 102 range persisted about once a day. The team wouldn't consider releasing Lilli until she was fever-free for at least 48 hours.

When Lilli's counts finally started going up more steadily and she had gone fever-free long enough, the team said that we could go home. For months, this was what I had been praying for. Lilli had made it to the end of her treatments, and she had lived to be able to go home for good. While there was that one scare with sepsis and the trip down to PICU, Lilli had rebounded well. Now we could go home again, like we had at the end of each of the other month-long rounds of chemo.

This time had a different feel. From December 12, 2014, until April 17, 2015, Lilli was at the mercy of the pediatric AML leukemia protocol, but she was now on her own. When each of the other rounds ended we knew that Lilli would get more chemotherapy to kill any remaining cancer cells that were hiding out, as the team described it. While chemotherapy was toxic and scary, I could count on its benefits to cure my daughter. Now Lilli's body would have no help to fight any remaining cancer. I could only pray that the chemo had killed off the cancer cells and had cured her.

We went through a few hours' worth of discharge paperwork, picking up prescriptions from the hospital pharmacy, and packing up the remainder of Lilli's things into plastic tubs and bins. It took a while to leave the hospital, but it was well worth the wait. What were a few more hours when Lilli had been in the hospital the better part of four straight months? I packed everything in LouAnne's van, and LouAnne headed out with Lilli while I returned the cart to the 9th floor unit. Before I could get out of the hospital, I got a call from one of the home health suppliers regarding our insurance.

How in the world can they call me this quickly? I haven't even left the hospital, and I'm already being harassed by folks for money. I guess this is what my future will be like: trying to figure out how to pay bills while being harassed by hospitals, pharmacies, and medical suppliers.

The issue was around our previous insurance policy that we had five years earlier, and it appeared to someone out there that we had two health insurance policies that were redundant. "No, I can assure you that I only have one insurance policy. No, that's an old policy. No, I don't even work for that company anymore. Yes, I'm telling you the truth, and my daughter needs this prescription to stay alive," I said. Once I convinced the vendor that I was telling the truth, they agreed to send over the person who would train us to use some of the home health products that we would need to use to maintain Lilli's central line.

Lilli rode home as she had done the previous rounds, riding the 30 minutes from Winston to Greensboro, and she was welcomed with a huge banner on our front porch. Amelia and Collin had worked on a "Welcome Home Lills" banner with crayons, markers, and colored pencils. "Lills" was Amelia's nickname for her sister. Together, they were Lills and Amils. While we didn't announce her return to the world, we wanted to make sure to celebrate her returning home for good this time. I went to our favorite bakery down the road and ordered a raspberry lemon cake with "#LilliSTRONG" written on it in icing, and the family celebrated with cake and board games.

Going home for good didn't mean cutting our ties with the hospital, however, as Lilli still had to go back regularly for blood draws and labs and check-ups with her doctors. It wasn't too long, merely a few days, before we went back for a check-up. After a good check-up and blood counts that continued to improve, Lilli's team said that they felt comfortable removing her central line. This was great news for us because it meant that we could stop flushing her central line every day she was home.

We left home one Tuesday morning in April for surgery. The experience of having Lilli's central line surgically implanted back in 2014 was one of shock and fear of the unknown. The extraction of her line was totally different. We had gotten to know the surgeon a bit better, and the surgery would take place in the main outpatient surgical suite, a space that seemed to be designed with the patient and patient's family in mind. We checked in at a reception desk, waited for them to call Lilli's name, and went back to a pre-op space where they started an IV and prepared Lilli for the procedure.

When they wheeled Lilli out of the prep room, LouAnne and I went back out to the waiting area where we watched a screen with patients' initials and ID numbers. We could watch for Lilli's ID and tell when she was having the procedure, when she was in recovery, and when she was finished. When they finished with the procedure, the surgeon called me and LouAnne to a small consultation room where she described the procedure and how well Lilli had done throughout the surgery. Then they called us back to a recovery area where Lilli was waiting for us. Lilli was a little groggy, and she had a bandage over the incisions where the line was extracted. The bandage covered the scar that Lilli will have the rest of her life.

In the parlance of the pediatric hematology-oncology team and the *Beads of Courage* program, Lilli had earned her *Purple Heart Bead*, a signature bead that marked the end of her treatment. We would check in with the child life team at Lilli's next clinic appointment to pick up this crowning achievement in Lilli's necklace. The child life specialist said that Lilli had also been selected for a special bead in the *Beads of Courage* program. Lilli would be able to sketch out a few thoughts for a custom-designed bead, and bead artists could sign up to make Lilli's--or another patient's--bead design.

Driving Lilli back home to Greensboro, I was full of hope. After the anesthesia wore off, and after a long nap, Lilli was back to her old self that afternoon. Amelia and Collin came home from school, and they could celebrate with the rest of us Lilli's wrapping up her treatment and the removal of her central line. Aside from Lilli's peach fuzz of hair and the mask that she was advised to continue to use, she looked like any other sixth grade girl again.

LouAnne and I could begin to get back to normal with our marriage and our careers. We could finally sleep in the same bed again and begin piecing together our family of five's daily and weekly rituals. We could bid adieu to LouAnne's parents and thank them for all they sacrificed to help us through our ordeal. I was thankful to have lived through the scariest four months of my life, yet I was frightened by the unknowns of being the father of a cancer survivor.

Appendix [Not That One]

Having faith in Lilli's recovery, LouAnne and I had RSVP'd to two of my former students' wedding in Durham a few weeks after Lilli's being discharged for good. The day before the wedding, LouAnne was not feeling well. She thought it was some stomach bug that would pass, and she said goodbye to her mom and dad as they drove off to go home to Middle Georgia. They had sacrificed themselves for months to look after our home and kids, and they deserved to get back home. That evening, with our family of five at home by ourselves, LouAnne had a fever and still an upset stomach. She tossed and turned in the bed, not able to sleep.

The next morning, LouAnne felt a little better but was not well enough to go to the wedding. I decided to go to the wedding solo, even if it meant some people might not believe me when I said that LouAnne was at home sick. I imagined that people would assume that we'd had some argument and that she had refused to go with me. "Sure," they'd think, "she's not well…" while believing that we were just like the statistical cancer parents. A couple who go through a family medical crisis like this are more prone to split up.

The wedding was industrial chic and picturesque, in an abandoned warehouse building in an industrial part of Durham, the backdrop you'd expect for artists and designers' weddings. I enjoyed seeing some of my former students and other university colleagues, and I think most believed me when I said that LouAnne was sick. Many of them had kept up with Lilli's story on Facebook and were curious to know how Lilli was doing. I did my best to answer questions, but I was still new to this. It would be months before I had my pat answers to the questions about Lilli's health. It didn't take long for me to avoid saying words like cancer-free, though, as I felt like there was no way to know for sure.

How would anyone know if he's cancer-free? Am I cancer-free? Do I know for certain there are no cancer cells hiding in my body? Could anyone know for certain?

When I got home that night LouAnne was still in pain, and it was unbearable. She said that she needed to get to the emergency room, which left us in a quandary. How could I drive her to the emergency room, leaving Lilli at home alone with her siblings? I wasn't about to go sit in an emergency room where I could catch who-knows-what from perfect strangers and then bring it back home where Lilli could catch it, too. At least one of us had to stay healthy to take care of Lilli. LouAnne, in a pinch, drove herself to the emergency room, and one of our friends from church met her there to sit with her through the night. They did tests to discover that LouAnne had appendicitis and needed to have her appendix removed the next morning. Luckily her appendix did not rupture, but there she was in a hospital without me since I was home with our kids.

Here we've spent four months in the hospital with Lilli, and we can't catch a break. Within weeks LouAnne's in the hospital to have surgery?

I couldn't believe how unlucky we were, but at least we had friends who sat with LouAnne in the hospital, swapped off the next day, sat with our kids the following day, and gave me a ride to the hospital to pick up LouAnne when all was said and done. We had become masters of managing crazy schedules and medical crises.

Now we have bills from one hospital for Lilli's cancer treatments and four months in the hospital, and on top of that we'll have a bill for an appendectomy. There's no way we can pay all of these bills, but there's also no precedent for us to ask our friends to help us pay LouAnne's hospital bills. It's one thing to ask for help for our innocent child, but it's another thing to ask for help for an adult who should have health insurance and all. Even with all of our insurance we can't pay all these bills without help.

At her one month check-up in late April, a few weeks after LouAnne's appendectomy, Lilli was looking great. I was getting used to the rhythm of the clinic appointments after graduating from the inpatient hematology-oncology unit of the hospital. After checking in at the clinic's reception desk, we'd wait to be called back for vitals. Lilli would have her height, weight, and blood pressure checked in a small room before moving further down the hall to Miss Pat for blood draws. Without a central line, Lilli had her blood drawn through a finger prick. After Pat would draw enough blood for the small vials, we'd go back to the waiting room or straight to an exam room, where Lilli would be examined by one of the young interns or fellows working in the clinic before seeing the oncologist. Some days, the team would share the lab results on the spot in the exam room. When the lab was slower, we would leave the hospital to head home, not knowing how Lilli's marrow was doing. We'd await a late afternoon phone call from the oncologists to learn the lab results. Those were the days when I would become the most stressed and anxious, running through different scenarios in my mind, including the worst case of Lilli's cancer recurring.

That day in April was a good clinic day. Lilli's blood counts continued to increase and were on the low end of the normal range for her age. Dr. Russell gave her the all-clear to get out in public, and Lilli beamed with light and joy at this news. She could now go back to church and public spaces like stores and restaurants, but most importantly Lilli could finally go back to school. LouAnne and I both took her to that appointment while Amelia and Collin were in school, and we were both there to witness Lilli's ringing the bell at the 9th floor clinic. Lilli smiled from ear to ear as we took plenty of pictures to capture the moment for ourselves and to share on Facebook. We celebrated by taking her out to The Loop for lunch. For the first time since December, Lilli was able to go into a restaurant, sit down, and eat a meal.

6th Grade Celebration

....

Lilli missed the second half of sixth grade. She spent most of that time in the hospital, and when she finally returned home to our modest brick ranch in Greensboro she still wasn't allowed to go to school. Until that clinic appointment in April 2015, Lilli's immune system wasn't strong enough for her to go out into public spaces like shopping malls, restaurants, or her own school. It was just too risky, and I wouldn't have forgiven myself if I had taken her somewhere where she could've caught something like a cold, easy enough for my immune system to fight but potentially deadly for our Lilli. Lilli was allowed to be at home—in our family's own micro-biome with our own germs—or a few other places, like the hospital for her regular check-ups or the great outdoors, like walking around the neighborhood which she did from time to time.

While she was waiting for the green light to go back to school Lilli was assigned a homebound teacher by the county school system. We had taken her out of the hospital school's system and had re-registered her with our home county's system. Having a homebound teacher was a requirement for Lilli to stay in good standing with the system and to maintain her place in the magnet middle school. I'm sure there are great homebound teachers out there, but the one assigned to Lilli that year was not a good fit for her. He was a full-time high school teacher who taught in the homebound program to make some extra cash after working his regular schedule. By the time he got to our house in the late afternoon he had already worked a full day. Lilli did not get his best, and ultimately, he operated more like a courier for Lilli's homework than a proper teacher who could teach Lilli anything.

Lilli couldn't wait to get back to school. We pressed the Brenner oncology team to let Lilli go back as quickly as possible, and when Dr. Russell finally gave her the go-ahead in May, she had about two weeks of school remaining. If anyone's visited a middle school in the final two weeks of the year lately, then they probably witnessed some end-of-year testing and a lot of celebrations and rewards for jobs well done. Lilli didn't care that she might miss out on all the instruction. She desperately missed the middle school environment and wanted to sit in a classroom once again. A day before Lilli was able to go back, LouAnne, Lilli, and I jumped in the car and drove up to Brown Summit Middle School. We gave the school advanced notice that we would stop by for a quiet visit.

We got to the school and found Lilli's counselor Ms. Denny who showed us down the hall to a classroom where some of Lilli's closest friends were waiting. Lilli was wearing her industrial strength facemask, mostly as a sign to stay back and to be careful around her. Lilli's friends, though, wanted to know if they could give her hugs, which they did. While Lilli's mask concealed her mouth, her eyes told the story of a girl aglow from being around her friends outside the hospital for the first time in months. Lilli's teachers who were in their classrooms while the students were at lunch were beaming with pride, with a few tears in their eyes.

I held back my own tears as I watched teachers and students so moved by Lilli's return. Ms. Denny asked if she could touch Lilli's peach fuzz on her head, and Lilli said "yes." I couldn't resist touching her hair, myself, as it reminded me of when she was a toddler and started growing hair. There's something perfect about a newly grown head of hair with even strands all around. We didn't stay long at school that day, as Lilli mostly wanted to check in, turn in some homework, and check out her locker. "Lilli, stand next to your locker while I take your picture," I said, "That one's going on Facebook."

Lilli had returned to school just in time to miss the end-of-grade tests and to make it to the end-of-year awards ceremony. When I was in the Putnam County Middle School in the mid-1980s there were no such things as end-of-year celebrations or assemblies for parents and grandparents, no awards ceremonies, trophies, or medals. I recall getting certificates for things like honor roll, but there was definitely nothing like what schools in the Guilford County Schools district throw for their students and families.

Will there be awards for each subject? Perfect attendance?
Honor roll? I don't know, but I hope they call Lilli's name
at least once. She deserves to have something go her way.

While Lilli was in her first or second round of chemo the first
awards ceremony of the year took place. We would've gone to that
one had Lilli not gotten sick. We found out that the day of that
mid-year ceremony was the day the school shot the #LilliStrong
Katy Perry *Firework* video. That same day a group of Lilli's friends
came to visit her in the hospital and gave her a sense of how awards
ceremonies were run at BSMS. The girls said they were long and
drawn out, as lots of students were recognized for A-honor roll or
A/B honor roll, and there were a few special awards for students in
each subject and for overall excellence.

Lilli hadn't been back in school for more than a week or two when
the end-of-year event took place. LouAnne and I drove her to
school that morning and decided to hang out there before the
ceremony, which meant that we were early for the event. I walked
into the gymnasium, turned auditorium with folding chairs, and
had a sense of how emotional I might be that day. I asked LouAnne
if we could sit in the front row, figuring that fewer people would
see us there if we were to become emotional.

I took a seat near the far end of the front row of folding chairs, all
lined up in even rows facing the stage, and LouAnne sat next to
me. Even though I knew some of the parents I decided not to start
conversations and to remain focused instead on the floor and the
chairs in front of us at some distance. The teachers and staff would
sit in those chairs turned the opposite direction, facing us, the
audience of doting parents and other family members. While I'd

be able to shield my emotions from the people sitting behind me, the teachers would have a front row seat to watch the two cancer parents' reacting to whatever would transpire.

Grab your popcorn, teachers! I don't know what's gonna happen, and there might be some ugly crying here.

The teachers who faced the crowd included the school counselor who had visited Lilli several times and had delivered a few envelopes full of donations from parents, students, teachers, staff, and strangers. She had also helped us set up a wi-fi router that allowed Lilli to bypass the hospital's internet firewall so that Lilli could log into the school's online accounts. A few chairs down from her was Lilli's English teacher who had shared an inspiring picture of an owl perched on a fencepost on the school grounds when he left school one afternoon. There was the PE teacher who had made custom journal pages with owls for Lilli to write down her thoughts and the Latin teacher who orchestrated the Katy Perry *Firework* video with the entire school. And there was the principal, Mrs. Mott, who supported our family through the entire ordeal and had kept her promise to hold Lilli's place in the school despite not knowing if Lilli would ever be able to return to the classroom.

As a magnet school for advanced academics, Brown Summit was full of brilliant students who would be recognized for all kinds of academic excellence, and it took a while to go through all the accolades. More sixth graders got A Honor Roll than did not, and Lilli was one of the students whose name was called and who walked up to shake the principal's hand and pick up a certificate. After half the students' names were called, the remaining half of A

Honor Roll students were out of space. There were A LOT of bright kids in that class, and they had to shuffle uncomfortably to make room for more students to squeeze into the line. The awards continued with different academic teams' being recognized and for some of the top individual awards.

I settled into the rhythm of the ceremony, not dwelling on Lilli, but the teachers and students had cooked up a few surprises for her. They had already produced the video earlier that year, and that would've been plenty for our whole family for a lifetime. But they went above and beyond to honor Lilli that morning. The counselor had asked us earlier to share digital photos with her so that she could do something with them. I didn't know exactly what she had up her sleeve, but the school put together a hardcover photo album that the teachers signed, and Mrs. Denny presented it to Lilli that morning.

At one point in the ceremony, Principal Mott called up some of the girls from the school who asked Lilli to come back up to the front with them. These young women had spent the second half of the year collecting yellow, orange, and brown owl-themed fabrics and had sewn together a custom quilt with these fabrics that were donated by several fabric shops around town. Around the perimeter trim of the quilt these same girls hand wrote an inspiring piece that was all about perseverance in the face of cancer. And on the white backside of the quilt just about every one of the students and staff wrote encouraging comments to Lilli. I couldn't believe how thoughtful these middle school girls had been, when middle school is generally the phase of life when people become more petty and rude towards each other. These girls showed such kindness and compassion and had decided to work on this project all by themselves without prompting from the school.

For the school's part, they did not leave Lilli out of their thoughts. The principal and other staff invented an award for Lilli and another sixth-grade student who was fighting Crohn's disease. The BSMS Phoenix Award honored a student who had suffered some setback but had arisen from the ashes after this personal struggle. By the end of the ceremony Lilli had been called up front at least three or four times to be recognized for her strength in the face of her life-threatening leukemia.

I couldn't control my emotions. I started bawling my eyes out when they announced the Phoenix Award. I buried my face in my hands, and I shook uncontrollably. For once LouAnne was the one who kept her composure while I totally lost it. It's funny how that's happened throughout this ordeal. I've noticed how LouAnne and I have balanced each other's emotions and states of mind. When one of us has been weak the other one has been strong. I was a mess. I had been holding back all these emotions for months, and I couldn't stop the spigot once the water started flowing. I sensed that the teachers were also emotional, as many of us were taking stock of the flooring and our shoes and anything else that kept us from looking at Lilli. Lilli, on the other hand, was still solid as a rock. She smiled and enjoyed the quilt, the plaque for the Phoenix Award, and the photo book.

Walking in the 'Wood

....

Lilli had been home a month or so when I stepped on the scales.
We had invested in a few scales around the house because of Lilli's
recovery and the importance of keeping track of her weight among
all the other numbers. For the first time that I could remember my
weight topped 230 pounds. I weighed in at 232.6 lbs.

*WHAT?! How did this happen? How have I gained this
much weight over the years?*

I couldn't believe that I had let myself go so much. I had stopped
exercising years earlier, around the time I finished grad school, and
I had lived a sedentary lifestyle of long hours at work and lots of
television watching. I had spits and spurts of walking around the

neighborhood or playing some basketball over the years, but I was out of shape. I was also overworked, having chosen a career in architecture that came with long hours and high-pressure projects and deadlines. I looked in the mirror and saw a fat, middle-aged man, a disappointment to myself and a far cry from the fit man LouAnne had married twenty years earlier.

I had to do something about my weight and my overall health. For several months, I had been taking the pills prescribed for high blood pressure, high cholesterol, and high triglycerides. I had kept them in my toiletries bag that went back and forth with me to and from the hospital while Lilli went through treatment. I detested the thought that I'd be a pill-popper for the rest of my life, imagining an elderly version of myself carrying around a pill organizer full of a kaleidoscope of pills that would keep me on medicinal life support. There had to be another way to live.

Lilli had lived through the four month-long rounds of chemo and had been released from the hospital with a clean bill of health. While the team didn't perform a final bone marrow aspirate, the doctors said that they felt Lilli was well and healed. The words I did not hear were "cancer free." I never pressed the doctors about this, but I came to my own conclusion and perspective. I determined that no one can claim to be totally cancer free. The nature of cancer is one of working at such a microscopic level as to be secretive, sneaking up on people when they least expect it.

For me to declare myself cancer free I'd have to extract and test every cell in my body, at which time I'd be dead. When people ask if Lilli is cancer free, I'll say that there's no way to know for sure but that she is doing well.

Feeling that Lilli was indeed well, I started to tackle my own health and wellness. After growing up on sweet tea and drinking it daily for the better part of forty years, I gave it up. Cold turkey. My mother would roll over in her grave if she were to find out I swore off sweet tea. I also gave up soft drinks, again cold turkey. I made a half-hearted attempt at giving up coffee, my Achilles heel, but after a few days of severe migraines and thinking twice about that decision, I decided to give up sugar in my coffee without giving up the coffee altogether.

And then I did something so simple that it was nearly impossible for my out-of-shape self. I started walking around our suburban *Westwood* neighborhood. I didn't start with any plan, but I thought I could at least walk around the block once. LouAnne had been walking around the neighborhood and had a few different routes, one hillier than others. I started with a flatter route, down the hill, left at the stop sign, left at the next block, and back up the hill to our house. I wondered if it would be at all possible to improve my health to such a degree as to cease taking those pills. If possible, then I would do my best to make it happen, as the pills were like an albatross around my neck.

Wearing the least athletic clothes on the block, I walked like the caricature of a nerdy old professor, minus the glasses. I had some cargo shorts and some cotton t-shirts. I wore an old pair of Nike low top basketball shoes, not walking shoes, along with black dress socks. I must've been a sight to see. I decided to invest in some no-show athletic ankle socks, but I didn't know enough to shop for proper walking shoes or athletic clothes. The cargo shorts' pockets were perfect, or so I thought, for holding my phone, my source for music as I walked around the neighborhood. I tried wearing earbuds but found that the cord made it hard to keep the earbuds in my ears. After a few walks, I decided to take off the earbuds and listen to my music out loud. The neighbors would just have to put up with my taste in music.

I had added walking to my fitness regimen of yoga. I walked sporadically at first, benefitting from the longer days of late spring and early summer. The mature trees in our mid-century neighborhood shaded me in the late afternoons and evenings when I could sneak away from the house to go for a walk. One parent had to stay at home with Lilli at all times, so I walked by myself. At other times, LouAnne walked by herself. Exercise was a solitary activity for us cancer parents.

PCSD

Watching Lilli go through chemotherapy treatments was hard.
Being the parent of a cancer survivor seemed even harder. Most of
my friends and family would ask about how Lilli was doing. She
was still the emotional rock that she was in the emergency room
that first night in the hospital. Most people avoided the question,
"How are you, Travis?" If they had asked, then I would've told
them that I was fine. But I wasn't totally fine. I was the father of a
child who had a chance of a relapse, or recurrence of a life-
threatening cancer. I was the father of two other children who,
statistically speaking, had a greater chance of having cancer.

*This is like PTSD, at least what I think I know about it,
except my trauma is from cancer and not from war. Post
Cancer Stress Disorder…that's it! That's how I'll describe
the anxiety, the bad dreams, the late nights' sneaking into
Lilli's room to make sure she's still breathing, and the*

overwhelming fear that in a moment's notice the other shoe will drop and we'll be back in the hospital again.

So, when Lilli had a nose bleed one morning that July, LouAnne and I freaked out. A bloody nose could be anything from "oh, nothing but some allergies," to "low platelets as a sign of cancer's return." I jumped to the worst possible outcome, that Lilli's platelets were low and that her blood wasn't clotting properly. We asked Lilli what she wanted us to do, and she asked us to take her to the clinic for a blood draw. For additional income to help pay bills, I was teaching a summer studio. I had to teach my class that day, so it was LouAnne's turn to take Lilli to the clinic. LouAnne checked in with the team that morning, and they agreed that it was a good idea to check Lilli's blood. From the studio that morning I kept up with LouAnne's text updates. LouAnne said that while Pat was drawing Lilli's blood from a finger prick that morning, Pat commented on how Lilli's blood was flowing more quickly than normal.

That's not what I want to hear! If her blood's flowing more quickly, then maybe her platelets ARE low. Were we missing anything else? Did Lilli have any petechiae? Why didn't we notice something sooner?

Lilli saw the doctor and nurses at the clinic, and they examined her while the blood samples were processed by the lab. Since the team had to work Lilli into the schedule with all the patients who already had appointments, it was in the afternoon when the lab results finally came through and the team was able to call LouAnne, who was back in Greensboro with the kids by that time, with the numbers.

I was driving home from the studio when LouAnne got me on the phone. I was in the Westerwood neighborhood near campus and pulled over to the side of the road to talk to LouAnne who told me that Lilli's platelets were NOT down but were slightly up from three weeks before. The rest of her counts were up, too, all but two of them in the ranges of perfectly healthy 12-year-old girls. Her bloody nose could've been a result of allergies or one of the many different and new things Lilli was exposed to over the weekend.

After hanging up, I sat in the car with all the windows rolled up. I was shaking uncontrollably while squeezing the steering wheel. I looked around to see if anyone was near my car. Seeing no one, I looked up at the clouds through my sunroof and let out a primal scream of release. Tears of joy and relief flowed down my face.

AAAAAaaaaaaaah! Thank You God! Cancer might take my girl from me someday, but today's NOT that day.

Relief replaced anxiety. I could breathe again. Today was not the day for our lives to be turned upside down again. While that day could very well come in the future, I was trying to take the highs and lows in stride and pray that God would provide. That day God provided us with continued health and recovery for our precious daughter, some added peace of mind, and some measured optimism that Lilli would make it to her Make-A-Wish trip in August. We parents were shaken but not defeated. We celebrated by dressing up like cows and enjoying a free meal at a chicken sandwich chain restaurant.

The bloody sinuses came and went.

That day was a microcosm of my experience as a cancer parent. There was a point of crisis in the nosebleed, followed by an unplanned hospital visit. I went about my daily routine at work while stressing out over the lab results. After what seemed like an eternity, I got the news that Lilli was doing well. Then our family celebrated our continued lives together.

While I wanted to know the outcome, the end to the story, from the first minute of that crisis, I would not have traded the journey for the world. Every moment in my experience was important, and skipping to the end would've meant missing out on all the human interactions and connections we made along the way. We met doctors, nurses, and hospital staff of the highest degree. We experienced a pediatric cancer unit where race, ethnicity, gender and religion were of no consequence where healing was a concerned. We experienced the healing power of art and music and had front row seats to the best in humanity.

It's a pity that it took cancer for us to have this experience.

Summertime '15

There was Make-A-Wish for patients, but I wished that there were some kind of wish for the parents, mostly LouAnne, after watching everything that she had gone through. I thought about what LouAnne might dream about, and I decided that I'd reward her on her birthday with a music workshop by one of her idols, Lynn Kleiner, in Washington, DC. And then I did what a Make-A-Wish staffer would do: I contacted Lynn Kleiner, explained our family's story, and described how much LouAnne idolized her and learned from her. I asked Lynn if she'd be willing to host LouAnne for a private dinner or coffee or something like that during the workshop, and Lynn was most amenable to my request!

In the summer of 2015 we packed up the whole family and headed up to Washington, checked into the conference hotel, and set out to explore the small neighborhood surrounding the hotel. We even found one of the DC Cupcakes bakeries, not the main one, but a smaller franchise one. No matter, however, because LouAnne and the girls had fallen in love with the DC Cupcakes story on TV about the grown sisters who ran a successful bakery in DC. The following day, while LouAnne was immersed in workshops and classes about teaching pre-schoolers music, I took the three kids on a tour around the Washington Mall. We hit as many museums and monuments as we could pack into a single day. We took the DC Metro, which meant that Lilli was on public transit and in a petri dish of germs. If there were any doubts about Lilli's immune system, we all chose to ignore these doubts for the benefit of our sight-seeing adventure on DC that day, one of the highlights of our summer.

Lilli enjoyed many normal activities, including swimming, hanging out with her friends, going to the movies, joining the church youth group, helping out with the church's Vacation Bible School, and completing her summer reading assignments for seventh grade that summer. Within reason, LouAnne and I made sure that she had all the supplies she needed to enjoy a normal summer. I struggled to know where to draw the line and didn't want to create a spoiled child, but I also tried to make up for all her lost time by saying yes to most of her modest requests for clothes, games, and the like.

That summer, I kept a close eye on Lilli. Her oncologists wanted to see her every few weeks, and they stayed on top of what was going on within her bone marrow and blood. Outwardly, Lilli was gaining strength and endurance, but I worried about every sneeze, sniffle, bug bite, and cough, thinking that everything could be a sign that the leukemia had returned. At the same time, however, I wanted to push Lilli to exercise and to regain her strength. All three kids showed an interest in tennis, so I bought tennis racquets for the whole family. We found public tennis courts at the local high school as well as the park where our Sunday school class would have summer picnics. The kids and I started going out for tennis once or twice a week, and Lilli kept up with her brother and sister. Not that I ever doubted Lilli's emotional strength through her cancer treatments, but now I could see Lilli's physical strength in recovery.

Towards the end of the summer of 2015 we had some time to celebrate by going on our Make-A-Wish trip, or Wish Trip. The staff were quite happy that Lilli had not requested a Disney World trip, because Make-A-Wish had a formula down pat for Disney and there would have been no planning by our local North Carolina connections. Because Lilli wished to go see her cousins in the Florida panhandle town of Navarre Beach, our local team with Make-A-Wish could actually do some planning. They asked Lilli for a Top 10 List of things she would like to do while in Florida, and she had a few things on that list in addition to spending time with her cousins. She wanted to go to an aquarium where they offered swimming with dolphins, go on a dolphin cruise, spend time on the beach, and go to the local zoo.

Make-A-Wish volunteers and staff organized a reveal party at an aquarium near Charlotte, over an hour's drive from Greensboro. They limited the number of people we could invite to the reveal party, and we asked Lilli for her list of friends. We wanted to make sure that her grandparents, parents, brother, and sister were on the list, too. On the day of the reveal Lilli's friends' parents dropped them off at our house. We piled them into LouAnne's minivan and my microvan, and we headed off towards Charlotte. The girls in

172

my car listened to some pop music on the radio, including a new one by Taylor Swift, *Bad Blood*. I had not heard that song before, but the girls had all heard it by that time. I'm not sure what the lyrics were about, but the term *bad blood* summed up Lilli's condition when she was first diagnosed with leukemia.

At the aquarium, we had behind-the-scenes tours, explored the public portion of the facility, and then had a cake and reveal party in a private party room. The place was all decked out in a beach theme, and our family was treated like royalty. The person who had donated the money to make Lilli's wish come to life was also there. It was great to meet him and to snap a few pictures, but he chose to be a fly on the wall and to maintain some privacy. We would not have had Lilli's Wish Trip without his generosity.

After the reveal party, we had to wait a few weeks until our trip to Florida. We bought additional luggage and some travel gear, and our anticipation grew. It would be the first time any of our kids had flown on a plane. It was also the first time that the rest of the family had ridden in a limousine. We packed for several days in advance of the trip and then awoke around 3:30 in the morning to catch the limo in front of our house. It was a stretch limo that took us to the RDU airport, a bigger airport than Greensboro's. We got out at the airport and took some pictures to capture the memories. As early as it was when we got to the airport, there were short lines to get through security and make our way to our gate. When we got to the gate LouAnne said, "Could you believe that they drove us over here in a Barbie pink limousine??"

"What?" I replied, "That was pink? I didn't notice it was pink." It reminds me of that debate about the color of the dress on

Facebook. Was it white and gold? Or was it teal and pink? Was that limo really Barbie pink? The pictures didn't lie. It was pitch black when the limo arrived, and at the airport I wasn't thinking about the limo. I focused on the luggage and getting to and through security and totally missed the striking color of the limo.

LouAnne's brother, Danny, his family, and LouAnne's parents, Joe and Janet, welcomed us to Florida. We were there for Lilli's Wish Trip, and she was not near death, despite my fears to the contrary when I first heard the words, "Make-A-Wish." It was possible for a Wish Kid to live through the experience of a wish, and we were going to make the most of Lilli's trip and not worry about her health for a few days.

I'm torn between wanting the whole world to know that Lilli fought cancer and was still alive and kicking…and wanting to disappear into the background and not have anyone know anything about our cancer experience.

We followed LouAnne's family from the airport towards Navarre Beach where we checked in to a beachside condo rental, a palace to us. We had never rented a place like this on vacation, and the kids felt like royalty to have an eighth-floor condo with an upper-level balcony and an expansive and open living room and dining room. We had separate bedrooms for the girls and for LouAnne and me. Collin camped out on the living room sofa. Looking out from the balcony to the Gulf of Mexico and a narrow slice of white sand and green waters of the Emerald Coast of Florida, we would watch ships, beachgoers, wild dolphins, storm clouds, bright skies, and rainbows.

I was in the middle of an online yoga challenge during our trip to Florida, committing to post at least one pic of myself practicing a yoga pose each day. I practiced some yoga on the beach, a bit embarrassing for an overweight, middle-aged introvert like myself, but I did most of the yoga indoors in the beachfront condo. I hadn't lost much weight, but I was more in tune with my body than I had been in years. Watching Lilli, Amelia, and Collin enjoying the beach and the luxury of a family vacation made me want to get in shape that much more.

Early one morning we drove down the highway to the nearby Gulf Breeze Zoo. Although in central North Carolina we have a huge zoo, I enjoyed the smaller zoo where we could get a little closer to animals. Make-A-Wish orchestrated extra perks at each of the stops. At the zoo, this meant that the kids got extra food to feed some of the animals and some spending money for souvenirs from the gift shop. On most of our previous trips we had such tight budgets that we'd have to encourage our kids to skip the gift shop by saying, "we can't afford that." My heart was warmed by the sight of the kids' shopping for trinkets.

Another day we went for a dolphin cruise in Destin, where I observed thousands of people hanging out on sand bars, drinking, and partying in broad daylight, definitely not our scene. We were there for a scheduled two-hour cruise around the bay to follow several pods of dolphins, and the dolphins did not disappoint. We saw at least 20 or 30 bottle nose dolphins in the bay. The overall congestion of the bay and the folks who rode alongside our boat on their jet skis, jumping into the water to harass the wild dolphins, took away from the picture postcard experience.

We had our own chance to interact with trained dolphins up close and personal on a different day when we drove down the coast to the Gulfarium on Okaloosa Island. We had tickets to the aquarium and to a special pool where we would get to swim with dolphins. We didn't swim so much as we walked in a pool where there happened to be several dolphins. The trainers worked with our family and one of two dolphins in the pool. After some general instructions about how to act around the dolphin, we got to do a few tricks with the dolphin.

I wonder who's really the trained animal around here? It feels like I'm having to follow more directions than this dolphin. Did she really just say "kiss the dolphin?" Oh, and they volunteered the dad to go first? Once in a lifetime is plenty for me to swim with a dolphin. Anything for my family, though.

Another day we had a private party and butterfly release at the Panhandle Butterfly House. This was not at the top of Lilli's list of things to do, but it was probably the most special and personalized activity of the whole Wish Trip. The butterfly house was only a mile or so from our condo, near the end of the bridge that connected our beach peninsula to the mainland. Several sweet older ladies who ran the butterfly house planned a special event just for Lilli and our family. I got the impression that we were the first Make-A-Wish family who had ever visited their place because they went all out for us. They had a custom cake and gift basket for Lilli and some extra goodies for Amelia and Collin. We all sat around in a covered gazebo and enjoyed the cake and lemonade and ice water before heading out to the covered butterfly house for a butterfly release. I had never been part of a butterfly release, a fascinating experience for all of us.

The staff had a box of roughly 100 flash-frozen butterflies from a butterfly farm, and it was our job to warm up each butterfly before letting them go free inside the butterfly house. Inside the box were tiny wax envelopes the size of butterflies that the staff removed one by one, handing each of us one at a time. We then unfolded the envelopes and watched as the butterflies awoke, warmed up inside the hot and humid butterfly house, and then fluttered away to find places to perch. Some of the butterflies were slower to awaken than others, and those butterflies were the ones with which we created brief human-to-insect bonds. I was mesmerized as they rested on our hands, fingers, shoulders, arms, legs, and clothes. One butterfly in particular, a green, brown, and white-colored malachite, rested on Lilli's index finger for several minutes while she studied it intensely.

I reflected on our experience with butterflies at church. It was a tradition at Guilford College UMC to bring in a net-covered basket full of butterflies on Easter Sunday. The story of transformation from caterpillar to chrysalis to butterfly was used to illustrate the transformation of Jesus from crucifixion to tomb to resurrection. The connection between butterflies and our Lilli was not lost on me, either. She had been born a normal baby and had grown up to become a leukemia patient when cancerous cells overtook her body. She then went through a transformation involving chemotherapy and a change in her body's bone marrow before emerging from her chrysalis as a newborn butterfly of a girl.

Aside from scheduled activities, we spent some free time with Lilli's cousins and LouAnne's family, the main reason Lilli had chosen this wish in the first place. The cousins had several sleepovers, some at our condo and others at my in-laws' house down the road. We ate lots of seafood at restaurants we normally bypass due to cost. On the cheaper side, I couldn't get enough of Tommy's SnoBalls and Boiled Peanuts just across the bridge from our condo. Make-A-Wish, our anonymous donor, and the staff made Lilli's dreams come true. She had lived out her dream to fly to Florida and spend quality time with her cousins, and we all got the family vacation we could never afford.

Falling Into Running

After walking once or twice a week for several months back in Greensboro, I decided to give running a shot on the spur of the moment. Walking to the end of the driveway and past the magnolia tree and mailbox, I thought, "What's the worst that could happen? I could die, but what if I don't die?" I was willing to take the risk, starting on the downhill from our house, not the uphill in our neighborhood of rolling hills. I could feel my weight right away, as my gut wiggled, jiggled, and bounced up and down as I ran. The phone in my shorts danced around, too, and I moved it to my hand for safe keeping. Still wearing my old cotton t-shirts, cargo shorts, and basketball shoes, I couldn't help but feel like all my neighbors' eyes were on me as I bounded awkwardly down the street.

I managed to run from our driveway to the first intersection down the hill, less than a tenth of a mile. To my surprise I was still upright after that short bit of running. I took a break from running and started walking down the street, past four, five, six houses. I walked to the next intersection and decided to try to run another block. I ran the next block, slow and steady, and I still had not died. I stopped and turned left at the stop sign, looking around to see if anyone else was approaching. The coast was clear, so I walked to the next intersection, turned left and continued around the block counterclockwise back to our street.

The downhill route from our house had flipped around to become a mountainous trek back home. I leaned forward as I caught my breath, shifted my weight forward, and tried to find some leverage to walk up the hill. Coming around the bend in the road, I lifted my head to see the top of my roof and the rest of our house emerge from behind the grass and pine straw of our neighbor's front yard. Slowing as I passed the familiar magnolia branches, I high-fived our mailbox, stopped in the driveway, and exhaled in exultation.

I did it! I'm not dead, and I'm going to try to run again next time. I want to live to see my daughter, correction, my whole family(!) grow up together.

After catching my breath and turning off my music, I walked up the steps to the side door to the kitchen. LouAnne, chopping veggies on the cutting board, noticed the extra sweat rolling down my face and drenching my clothes. "What did you do?! If all that sweat is from walking around the block, then you need to see the doctor."

"I ran a little bit," I replied.

"You're gonna kill yourself, Travis! I can't have you die on me after all we've gone through. Please be careful, and don't run anymore," LouAnne begged.

Despite LouAnne's pleadings, I kept running around the neighborhood. I had survived the first run in the neighborhood, and I was determined to continue running...or die trying. The pain and exhaustion from running were temporary compared to the medications that I imagined to be a life sentence. I was running for my life.

The combination of running, yoga, and cutting out sugar in my diet led to fast results. I was shedding pounds quickly, and in a matter of months I had sub-200 pounds in my sights. It had been nearly 15 years since I saw any weight lower than 200 pounds, and I didn't want to jinx my chances of getting there. I kept these fitness gains to myself for a while, except on my Instagram account, where I had found accountability through the monthly yoga challenges and the private training group set up by my virtual coach Cindy. My secret affair with running would have to wait a while before I'd announce it to the world.

Thirteen

In the fall of 2015, my whole family prepared for the start of school. I was starting my sixth year as a full-time assistant professor at UNC Greensboro, having put off my promotion and tenure review for a year due to personal exigency, a policy put in place for people in situations just like mine. Instead of putting together my tenure dossier in the spring while Lilli was a patient in the hospital, I could wait for a quieter spring the following year. Lilli, Amelia, and Collin were getting ready for the start of 7th, 5th, and 2nd grades, and LouAnne was getting back into her pre-schools and daycares, finally able to return to a fuller schedule of music classes after cutting back to three days a week the previous winter.

Lilli was happy to get back to the classroom as a seventh grader at Brown Summit Middle. After cancer had stolen away half a year of normalcy from her sixth-grade year, Lilli was back. With support of the hospital school and teacher, Lilli's home school, and technology that kept her connected, Lilli had not missed a step. She finished off the previous year with straight As and remained on track with her cohort of friends.

Lilli's 13th birthday was that September, about 9 months after she was diagnosed with leukemia. Our family made an impromptu trip to Georgia for her birthday weekend, where we saw friends and family who had been praying for Lilli and anxiously waiting to see her. We invited our extended family to celebrate with us at a local restaurant in LouAnne's hometown. It was like a family reunion for both sides of our family, as 25-30 people traveled from near and far to see Lilli. When family members heard about Lilli's diagnosis, some of them wanted to see her but also didn't want to make her sick while her immune system was compromised. With the birthday luncheon in Georgia, these folks could finally see Lilli without fear of killing her.

We followed that Georgia trip with another birthday party in North Carolina catered by the owner of the local Zaxby's restaurants. Why would a Zaxby's owner donate food, drink, and Zax-cessories to Lilli's party? If you had visited Brenner Children's Hospital when Lilli was in her third and fourth rounds of chemo you would have found Lilli eating Zaxby's boneless buffalo wings or chicken strips nearly every day. Earlier in her treatment it was Panera Bread soups and Starbucks hot chocolate, but by the later rounds Lilli craved Zaxby's. A visitor to the hospital made a call to a family member in Zaxby's corporate office, and that family member made a call to the local owner who contacted us and offered to cater Lilli's party. He came with chicken strips, chips, salads, wings, celery stalks, dressings, condiments, and sweet tea.

For Lilli, Amelia, and Collin he brought Zaxby's uniforms, complete with shirts, nametags, and hats, as though our kids could go straight to work for him. Lilli blushed from all the attention, but she was all smiles at the sight of the food and gifts.

Lilli invited some of her close friends from school and church to enjoy the chicken dinner and to stay for cake and a group art project. Lilli and I had planned a painting exercise for everyone, and they enjoyed painting in acrylics on small canvases. We set up a makeshift art studio in our kitchen and dining room, and I provided a demonstration by painting a sketch portrait of Amelia that still floats around our house. Lilli painted a tree, divided down the middle, with a winter half and a fall half. Lilli's painting still hangs in our laundry room beside a painting that says "#LilliStronger" and a still life done by Amelia that night.

On the outside, Lilli appeared to be a normal teenager who fit right in with her friend group. Her hair was still growing back, curlier and darker than before. Before cancer, Lilli had long, straight, thick, light brown hair. The nurses and CNAs told us that chemo would most likely change her hair. We had heard similar stories from friends and family members who had gone through chemo. It was no different with Lilli, who looked different than before cancer. She continued to look healthier, but each month reminded me of how close we still were to the cancer diagnosis that wasn't even a year old. I would stress out for several days leading up to one of Lilli's check-ups at the clinic, and for several months there were excellent blood counts. Lilli even grew two inches and gained 15-20 pounds from January to September 2015.

Lilli's doctors were pleased with her progress and started talking about her restarting the course of vaccinations. Chemotherapy had wiped out Lilli's immune system on a monthly basis for four straight months. This process had also wiped out all the immunizations that she had developed, either by contracting something or from shots at the pediatricians' offices. Lilli's immune system was like that of a newborn baby, and she would have to undergo all those same vaccinations that she had gotten when she was a baby, toddler, and growing child. Because Lilli was vulnerable to catching anything and everything, we had to be careful about whom we let into our home and where we took Lilli outside our home.

In late October 2015, Lilli was baptized. While I had prayed for her baptism, LouAnne and I let Lilli arrive at this milestone on her own without pressure from us. The day of her baptism was even more special as our family played special music during the church service. Lilli had taken violin lessons since kindergarten, and Amelia had taken tenor banjo lessons for several years. The girls played their instruments, I played my low whistle, and Amelia's banjo teacher, Scott, played guitar. We played several tunes during the service, attended by our whole family, LouAnne's parents, my dad, and my Aunt Barbara. I felt some relief knowing that Lilli had made a commitment to her faith and to her God, in case the cancer was to return and take her life.

Beyond those milestones of birthday and baptism, our family got back into our groove of work, home, school, church, scouts, music lessons, homework, weekends, cooking, cleaning, other chores, arguing, talking back, teen angst, and other normal activities. Lilli returned to the Greensboro Symphony Youth Orchestra after taking off nearly a year. She had performed with the orchestra only once, shortly before her diagnosis, before having to drop out. Lilli and I cultivated a Sunday afternoon ritual in which I would take her to orchestra practice at UNCG's music building and then walk down to Tate Street Coffee for the weekly Irish music session. It had been a while since I had regularly attended a session.

This is too good to be true. Lilli's orchestra practice coincides with the weekly Tate Street Irish session. I've never had such a good excuse to play the pipes and whistles every week, and Lilli has jumped right back into the orchestra. We are blessed.

Fall had arrived. While Thanksgiving stirred memories of the previous year's concerns about Lilli's cold sores and her loss of energy, I tried to focus on the positive and on the anniversary of Lilli's cancer diagnosis, her "cancer-versary." Through Facebook and MealTrain, I requested that our friends and family members wear their blue, purple, owls, and #LilliSTRONG shirts and wristbands to mark the occasion. Surviving for a year post-diagnosis was a milestone for Lilli, and I wanted her to see the positive support and energy from our community.

The night before Lilli's cancer-versary, Lilli and I rode to Winston-Salem for a concert, but not just any old concert. We went to hear the album-launch for Colin Allured, the red-headed music therapist who taught Lilli the baritone ukulele in the hospital. He had left the hospital for a full-time career as a musician and singer-songwriter. He wrote all the songs on this new album, and he performed as a veritable one-man-band on guitar, percussion, and vocals that night. Lilli and I saw a lot of familiar faces there, including doctors and nurses who, like us, had come to support our friend from the children's hospital.

During intermission, Lilli and I bumped into Dr. Wofford, the oncologist who had first diagnosed Lilli a year earlier.

"We were in a totally different place a year ago," I said.

"Oh, hey, Lilli. Good to see you," Dr. Wofford responded.

While I was proud of Lilli's progress and pleased that we were not in the hospital, I felt like I was tempting fate to brag about how far we had come in a year. In my irrational, paranoid moments I felt like the cancer cells could sense my pride and joy in Lilli's success and would respond by saying, "Oh, yeah, we'll show you." This paranoia kept me on pins and needles, constantly looking for signs of cancer when I looked at Lilli.

The day of Lilli's cancer diagnosis anniversary was a Sunday. At church, we were met with a sanctuary full of people wearing blue and purple and owls in honor of Lilli. Lilli's youth minister, Robert, made a point of honoring Lilli, saying that she was a walking miracle to have survived an aggressive cancer that tried to take her life a year earlier. At school the following day, Lilli's friends wore the same colors and celebrated her survival. And at Amelia's and Collin's elementary school—Lilli's old school—the teachers and classmates also wore their colors and #LilliSTRONG t-shirts. I loved seeing the support that our community showed Lilli those days, and I hoped and prayed that she would continue to recover and thrive amidst the possibility of a relapse.

Running for My Life

....

I had been running for a month or two in my un-athletic gear in our neighborhood when I decided to invest in some better gear. I drove the short distance to TJ Maxx and checked out their athletic wear section.

Boy, clothes have come a long way since I played high school sports! So many options…where do I start?

Jonathan, one of my runner friends from church said that I should get some wicking clothes and described the concept of wicking to me. I went home and Googled, "What is a wicking shirt." It's embarrassing how little I knew about proper athletic gear, but I didn't own a single wicking thing. I found a few cheap shirts and pairs of shorts, along with a pack of no-show running socks, and I was half-way there.

Jonathan also suggested that I get fitted for proper running shoes. I was just waking up to the concept of running shoes. "Like, there are different types of sneakers designed for running? I thought they were all pretty much the same and that I should just go for shoes that feel good on my feet," I told him. Instead of getting fitted by a specialty running store at the time, I went instead to a cheaper shoe store and just looked for any shoe that said "Running." I found a shoe that was on sale and that felt good on my feet, and I paid what I thought to be an exorbitant amount of money for a pair of shoes, around $70. These shoes completed my first semi-official running outfit, and I was ready to conquer the world of running.

I ran around my neighborhood for a few more months in my new outfit, trying to figure out what my mile pace was. If you had asked me two years earlier what "mile pace" even meant I wouldn't have known. But I had heard some of the runners at church talking about pace and such. I failed to make a connection between technology and running at that time, so I got in my car and drove around my neighborhood, some of the same routes that I had been running, and clocked how far they were on the car's odometer. I found a one-mile route that I had run a number of times, and I decided to run that route consistently and use my phone's stopwatch feature to time how long it took me to run a mile. I ran the route enough to figure that my mile pace was somewhere around 9-10 minutes per mile. I had no idea if that was good or bad. I guessed that it wasn't world class, but I wasn't sure what to expect as a beginning runner.

At a holiday party, some of those same runner friends from church were talking about their training plans, shoes, routes, accessories, and races. I now know that these are the kinds of things that all runners like to talk about, but at the time it was a whole new world to me. Andy, an experienced runner with multiple marathons under his belt, was talking about being fitted for new running shoes. It sounded to me like some kind of pseudo-science, but it made perfect sense at the same time.

Was I a pronator? Supinator? Was I a heel-striker? Mid-striker? These were all new terms to me, and I thought they were reserved for real runners.

But I'm still not a "real runner," and I don't want to embarrass myself by going to a running shoe store to be fitted. I need to run more miles before I'll know enough to be fitted for a shoe.

Jonathan talked about the running app on his phone. "They make apps for that, too? I should've known there'd be apps for that," I said. He showed me the app that captured the route he had just run earlier that day, the pace, the mile splits, calories burned, cadence, and more. It was something like six miles.

"That's as many calories as a Big Mac," he added.

6 miles?! I'll never be able to run 6 miles. I'm happy just being able to run 2 or 3 miles. But an app like that…I could stop driving around the neighborhood and instead use that app to calculate my time and distance. I could once and for all tell how fast I can run a mile.

I was hooked! I went home that night and downloaded the app on my phone, ready to use it the next time I ran. I could finally tell for sure how far and how fast I was running. The treasure chest was unlocked.

Andy and Jonathan suggested that I just go ahead and sign up for a race and start training. "Start with a 5k. There are plenty of them around here, and it's pretty easy to train for that distance if you can already run a mile," Andy advised.

"If you can run one mile, then you can run two. If you can run two, then you can run three," Jonathan said. Jonathan and Andy advised me to keep it slow and steady and to increase my mileage incrementally, around a 10% increase per week.

Over the 2015 Christmas holidays we were in Georgia visiting family, and I kept running, for the first time around the downtown of LouAnne's hometown of Milledgeville. I sat in the BlackBird Coffee shop, enjoying a latte plus a large ice water, after one of my runs. I had finally succeeded in running a 5k, or 3.1 miles, around the antebellum capital of Georgia without stopping. This was a big deal for me.

Why not sign up for a 5k race back in North Carolina? And where do I go to find a race?

From the coffee shop, I searched for upcoming races in NC on my phone. I found a plethora of races once I clicked on the proper database. And there it was, the perfect race for my very first 5k: the "Let's Lick Leukemia 5k" in a town about 1.5 hours away from home. It was organized by a high school student for a service-learning activity to raise money in honor of one of her friends who had fought leukemia. How could I not run that race? With sweat pooling on my metal bar stool in the Blackbird, I signed up for the 5k on the spot.

Back in North Carolina I trained a little harder, knowing that my first 5k was coming up. I was more fit and had lost around 30 pounds since the summer. About a week before the 5k, however, I got a cold that almost knocked me out of the race. I went to see my doctor and asked if he thought I could run a 5k in my condition. He didn't say "no," but he also didn't say "yes." By race day I had improved just enough that I felt comfortable going for it.

The race was on a Sunday afternoon, and I drove the hour and a half by myself after church that morning. There was snow on the ground, and I had by that time learned enough about running gear that I had cold weather running clothes and accessories. The race organizers had let participants know to bring photographs of leukemia patients, survivors, or angels, and I obliged by taking a few pictures of Lilli that I taped to one of the posters they had hanging off the edge of folding tables next to the starting line on the track.

This homegrown, high schooler-organized, small-scale 5k was a tiny race. There might have been 25 or 35 participants, tops. The race course was the same as the high school cross country team's course and seemed a little convoluted to me. I asked if the course would be marked, and the organizers—the high school student and her mom—said that it would be marked, with volunteers at most of the turns. Though few in number, runners and walkers of all ages showed up, including a few families. I was one of the older runners.

When we started there were a few fast runners who were together, a competitive family who took off like rockets. I was one of a handful of runners in a pack trailing that fast family, and we followed them down a wooded trail after two twists and turns. After a while, another runner and I stopped and looked at each other. I asked, "Are we going the right way? This wasn't advertised as a trail race." About that time, we turned around to see one of the volunteers' flagging us down to say that we were off course.

The fast runners in front of us had already jumped a creek and headed out of sight up another hill in the woods. A few of us turned around to return to the official course. By that time there were about 10 to 15 runners who had passed us because they stayed on course. I took a moment to walk a bit, compose myself, re-insert my earbuds, turn on my music, and start running again. I resigned myself to finishing at the back of the pack as I had gotten off course, lost five minutes, and been passed by others.

I can't quit now. Lilli didn't quit when she was weak and bald. So what if I don't win this race! I'm gonna finish as strong as I can, no matter what.

I started running and passing runners and walkers as I went. When I made it around the first of two loops on the high school grounds, I guessed that there were still four or five runners in front of me. I kept up my running, repeating the mantra "don't give up," over and over. When I got closer to the end of the second of two loops, I couldn't tell if anyone was in front of me or not, as some people were still on their first loops and others were running laps around the track where we finished.

Reaching what I thought was the finish line, I looked at the race organizers who were manning the tables where they had taped the posters. They looked back at me and said, "You won!" and handed me an envelope with a hand-written note: "First Place Male." I couldn't believe that I had won. A minute or so later a woman runner who, like me, had gotten off track, crossed the finish line and got an envelope for first place female. When I looked at my phone app I discovered that I had run more than a 5k. Instead of running 3.1 miles, I had run over 3.5 miles in around 33 minutes, about the slowest I had run in months.

I didn't quit. In perhaps the most unconventional race I've ever run, I won first place overall in a 5k. This was beginner's luck, one might say. One of my runner friends from church later said, "It's nice to win a place in your age group."

"Oh, I won first place overall with a time of 33 minutes," I clarified.

He shook his head and said, "The Lord works in mysterious ways."

I nodded. There's no way that my time would've won any other 5k I've ever run or considered running.

What was in my envelope for being first place male runner? It was a $25 Starbucks gift card. As a committed—some might say addicted—coffee drinker, I felt like they had read my mind. I got the perfect award for the less-than-perfect 5k, and I felt great to have been able to honor Lilli by putting her pictures up on the posters with the other photos. I took it all in, walking a few laps around the track and taking selfies to post on Facebook and Instagram. A woman who walked and finished the race while I was cooling down struck up a conversation and said, "Oh, I see you won? Congratulations! I could tell you're a real runner by how you look. You look like you know what you're doing."

Did she just call me a real runner? Am I a real runner? Does this really count since I won on a fluke?

I oscillated between having confidence in my running abilities and feeling like an imposter in this new world of running. Nevertheless, I was fully committed to claiming my coffee prize. On the long drive home that afternoon, I couldn't resist stopping at the nearest Starbucks on I-40 and getting my usual, a grande latté, hot. There was no oscillating there.

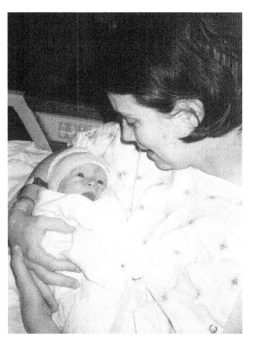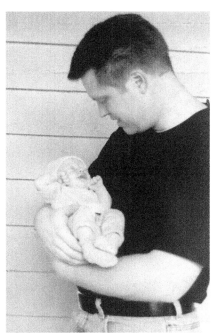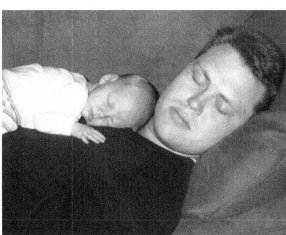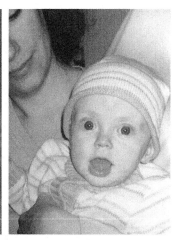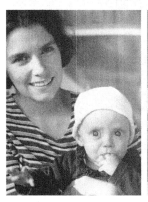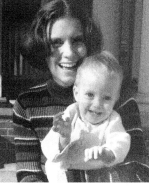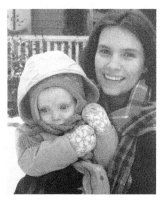

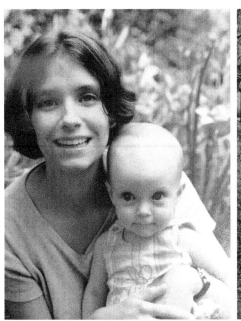
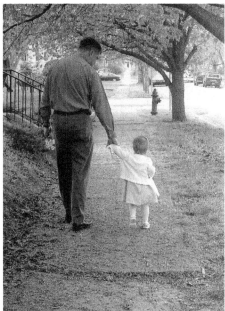
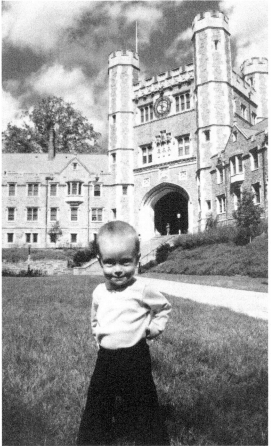
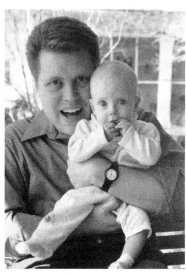
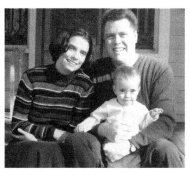

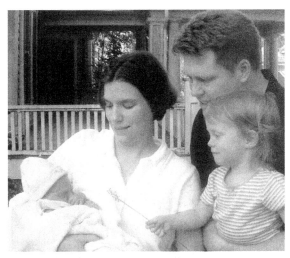
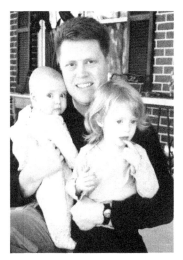
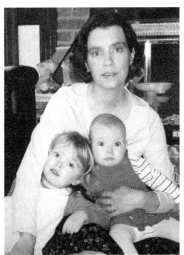
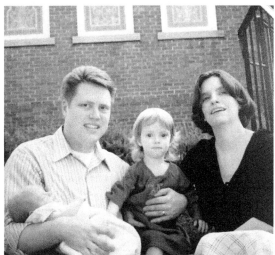
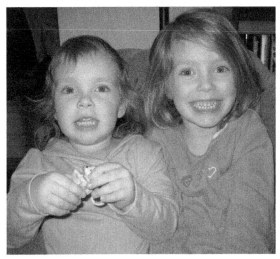
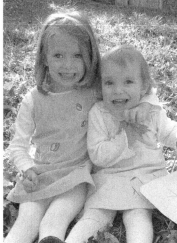

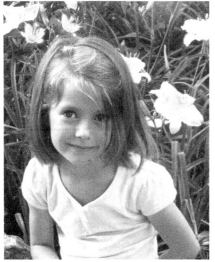
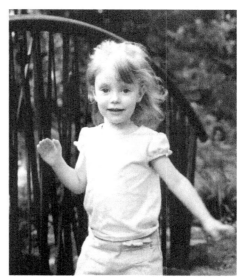
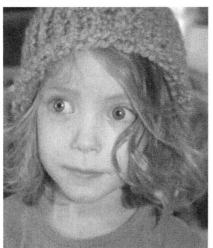
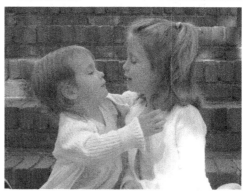
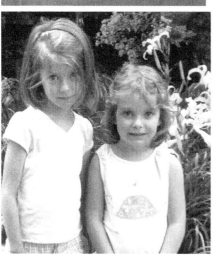
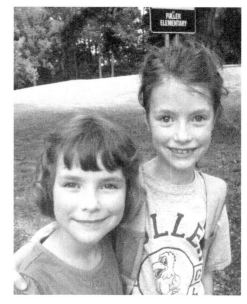

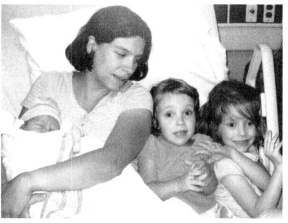
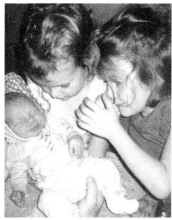
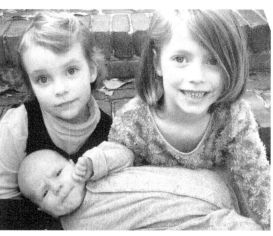
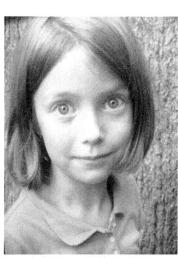
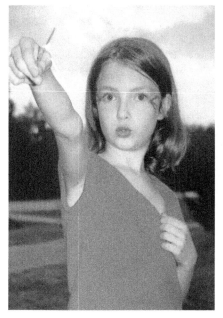
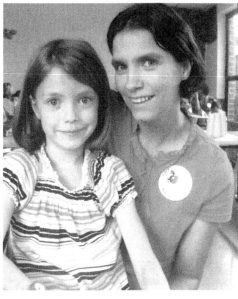

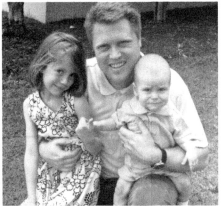

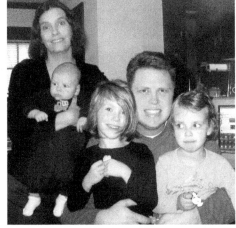

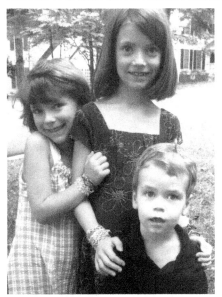

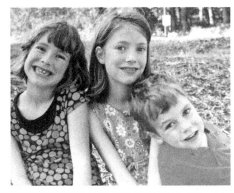

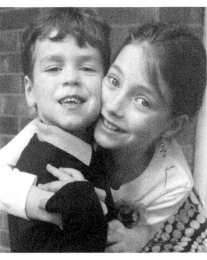

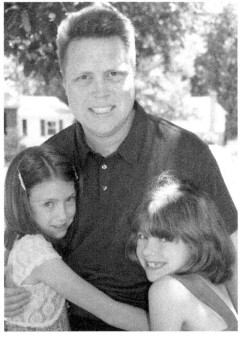

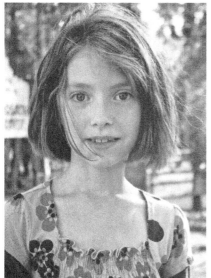
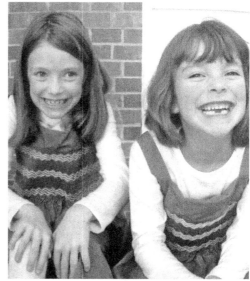
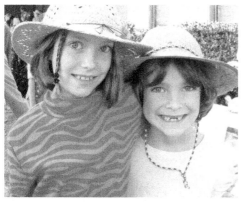
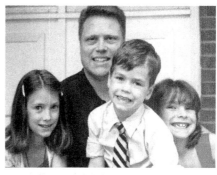
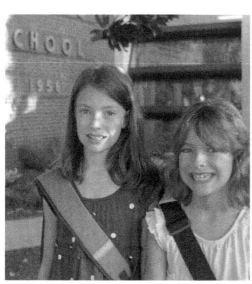
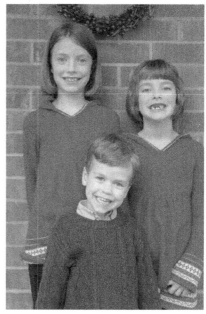

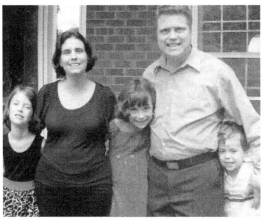

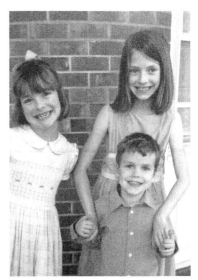

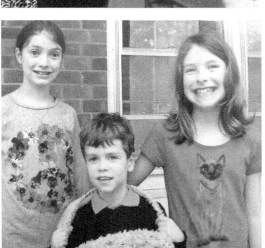

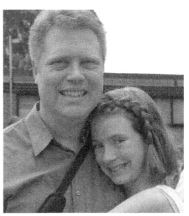

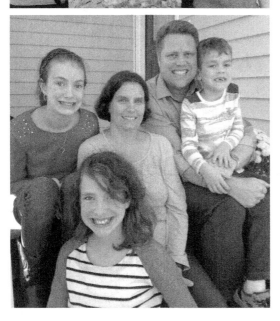

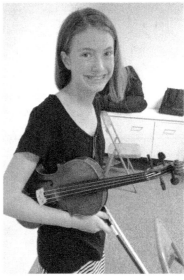

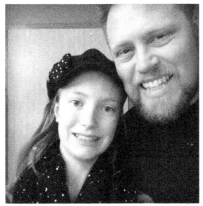
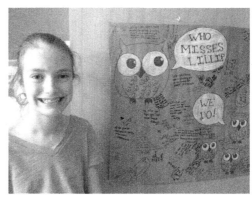
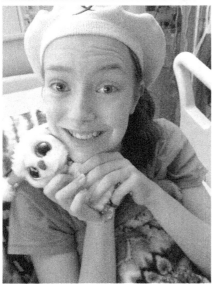
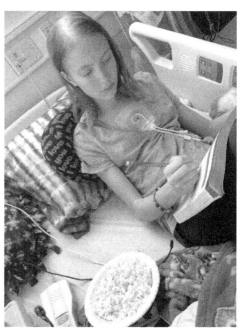
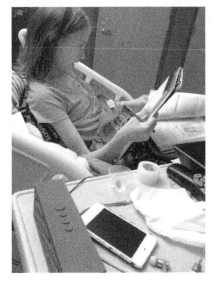
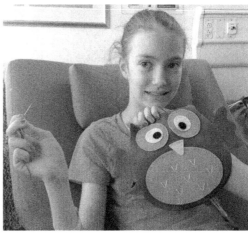

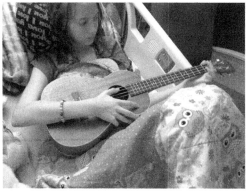
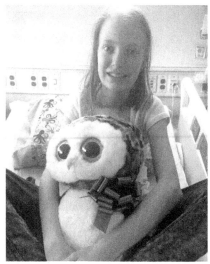
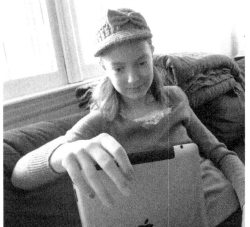
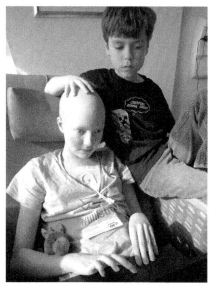
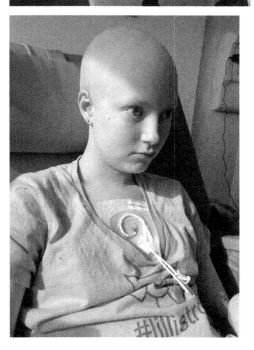
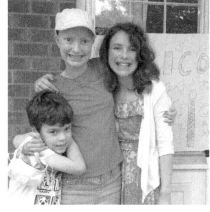

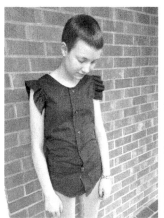 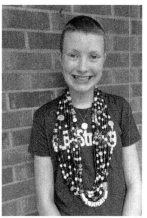 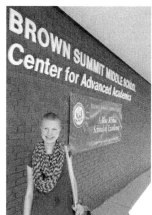

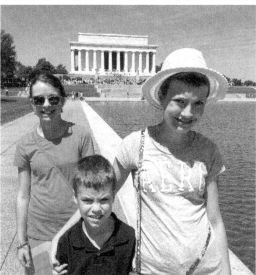 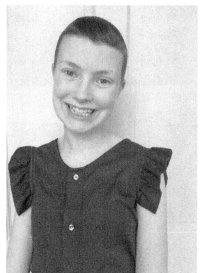

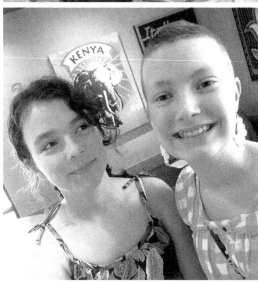 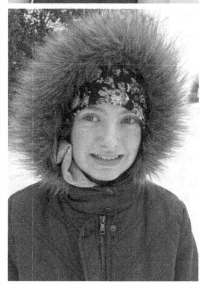

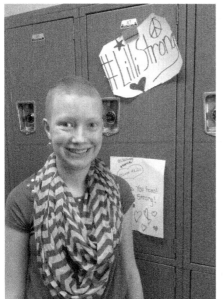
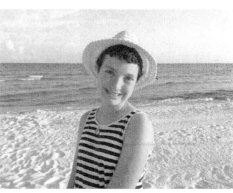
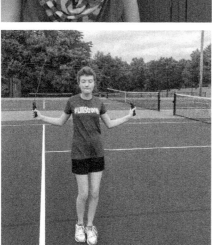
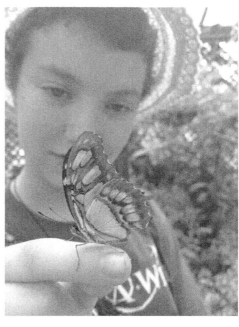
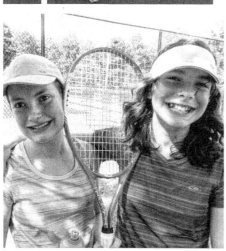
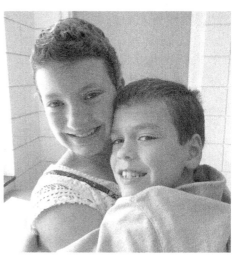

Part Two

The Return

When we went to Georgia to visit family over the Christmas and New Year's break, Lilli had been fighting some kind of cold or virus for a few weeks. When people asked how she was doing I would say that she was doing okay but that she was fighting something, either a cold or allergies. She was definitely better than she was the year before, I kept saying. I kept a close watch on her the entire trip, however, and I worried every time she coughed or sneezed. I didn't know what a perfect recovery from AML looked like, but I had my doubts that Lilli was recovering as necessary.

For weeks after we returned from our trip to Georgia, I had a gut feeling that Lilli's cancer had returned. I had worried all fall and into the winter as her blood counts, particularly her ANC, had not rebounded as strongly as I thought they should. While the oncology team kept reassuring us of good-enough lab results, I could tell that something wasn't quite right. Her blood counts seemed to bounce up and down, mostly lower than normal ranges.

Shouldn't she have bounced back by now? Maybe they're right when they say it takes time. But I wish that she would recover faster or better than she has. I don't know what I'll do if her cancer returns.

There was one clinic appointment in late January 2016 when Lilli's ANC (Absolute Neutrophil Count), a measure of her body's ability to fight off infections, viruses, and the like, had dropped to 500 (a normal ANC is between 1,500 and 8,000). Lilli was neutropenic and at risk for catching all kinds of things, especially considering it was flu season. Lilli and I had waited a while that afternoon for her lab results. Waiting in the 9th floor clinic with a teenager was rough, because most of the distractions there, like the TV and play room, were oriented to younger kids. I worried why it was taking so long for the results, which eventually came hand-written on a post-it because the printer was down.

"ANC – 500"

A year earlier those letters and numbers would've meant nothing to me, but that day they were alarming. Kat, who had handed me the post-it, paused for a moment. I said, "Kat, she's neutropenic, right?!"

"Yes, she is," Kat replied, "We had the lab look at the cells under the microscope, though, and they look good." I couldn't just walk out of the clinic without further details, so Lilli and I walked back to the staff area. Kat asked us to bring Lilli in for blood draws more frequently during January and February, wanting to keep a closer eye on her. For most of those appointments Lilli's counts remained low; however, the clinic kept reassuring us that, upon looking at the cells carefully, Lilli was doing okay and that her body's white blood cells were probably fighting off the various bugs out in the world.

I asked the team if Lilli was still okay to go out in the world, despite her being neutropenic, and they cleared her. We were responsible for keeping a close eye on her, should she start to show signs of illness more serious than a cold or allergies. I continued watching Lilli, paying attention to every sniffle, sneeze, and cough, looking for any signs that she was not well. In the hospital, there was a safety net for our sick daughter, but at our home it was just a family of five with no life-saving medicine and no formal medical training. I kept looking for signs of Lilli's improving or declining.

OK, she's just fighting some kind of cold virus or allergies. This is just par for the course for someone who's rebuilding an immune system. At least the blood cells don't show a recurrence of leukemia under the microscope.

This is what I told myself to make it through each day, when in the back of my mind I was totally freaking out. LouAnne and I had lived through the worst news of our lives once already, and I braced myself for bad news again.

In spite of my gut feelings, I invited Lilli out for a run one day after school. Lilli had been running in PE and had clocked a mile at around ten minutes, and I wanted to see how she would do on my normal route near Guilford Courthouse Battleground. On that brisk afternoon, I drove the two of us the short distance from our house to the visitor's center parking lot, and we got out of the car to stretch a bit before heading up the greenway. I tried to tell Lilli to take it easy and to go slow, but she started running too fast at the start and soon had to stop and walk when we turned towards the cemetery. This was the same cemetery I ran past numerous times a week, the same cemetery where a gravestone with "HICKS" inscribed on it jumped out at me early one fall morning, the same cemetery where I had imagined potentially burying the daughter who was now walking alongside me. I couldn't tell her those thoughts, though, even as I wondered why she was struggling to run half a mile after running a ten-minute mile in PE.

Is she fighting a cold? Is that why she can't run very far? Has the cancer returned? Are leukemia cells taking over her body again?

After what turned out to be a one-mile set of running and walking intervals, Lilli and I returned to my car. She was exhausted but happy to have gone for a run with her Dad. I smiled as we took a selfie to mark the occasion of our first run together, but my heart was heavy with thoughts of cancer.

Lilli's labs a few weeks later were similar, still low, and the clinic staff continued to reassure us that the cells looked okay under the microscope. The team was evidently concerned about Lilli, however, because for the first time in over a year I got a call from Kat in the clinic in the middle of the day during a week when Lilli didn't have labs. I had to step out of a meeting to take the call. "Mr. Hicks, I'm just calling to check on Lilli and see how she's doing. Is she well enough to go to school and other places? How is her stamina? Have you noticed anything concerning you?" I wanted to scream that getting a phone call from out of the blue was pretty darn concerning. I was convinced that the team sensed something from Lilli's labs, a trend, a pattern, something that matched other historical patients with AML such that they could see something coming. To me it seemed like just a matter of time until the other shoe would drop.

Then one afternoon in late February 2016, the day after one of Lilli's subsequent clinic visits, our world was rocked yet again. I was about to leave campus for a meeting with a professor from NCA+T across town. He and I had been e-mailing back and forth about collaborating on a project. That project would have to wait because I never made it to that meeting. He and I wouldn't connect for over two years. Just as I prepared to leave the office and go out to my car I got a call with a Winston-Salem number.

"Mr. Hicks, this is Dr. McLean…"

With that I walked out the door and entered the vacant storefront next door to which I had a spare key. I couldn't take that call in an office full of my colleagues and students, as I knew that any call from him, the head of the pediatric oncology department, signaled that my fears had come true. I paced around that cold, empty space as Dr. McLean proceeded to tell me the news that I had expected for weeks. "We got a call from the pathology lab earlier today. They found some funny looking cells in Lilli's sample from yesterday. There's a good chance that the cancer has returned."

The rest of the phone conversation was a blur. I had to ask him to repeat some of the points he made. When I asked for a percentage, for his gut opinion, a chance that he was wrong, Dr. McLean said that there was perhaps a 25% chance that the cancer was not back, that the increase in white cells was due to some virus and not to the return of leukemia. "What happens if the cancer is back?" I asked. In a matter-of-fact tone—one that I'm sure he'd practiced and perfected over many years of breaking similar news to other fathers—he proceeded to summarize the protocol for an AML recurrence. Lilli would first receive more rounds of chemotherapy at Brenner to get her back into remission followed by a bone marrow transplant at Duke University Hospital, as Brenner did not perform pediatric bone marrow transplants.

I asked if we had to rush to the hospital for immediate labs and for Lilli to be admitted, and he said no, to come in on Monday for another bone marrow aspirate and blood tests. He suggested that we enjoy our weekend at home and not worry about any immediate danger to Lilli, as she had appeared to be fairly healthy while in clinic the day before. Whenever the team would suggest that we enjoy some family time at home, I suspected some ulterior motive. Was "family time" code for "enjoy your last few days with her at home while you can?" I tried to banish that thought from my mind, but I had been through enough scary phone calls that I interpreted all news through the scars from previous experiences.

While I held out hope for that 25%, I felt in my heart that the cancer had returned. I had the daunting task of holding myself together while driving the twelve minutes home to break the news to Lilli and the rest of the family that her leukemia could be back.

What do I say? How do I say it? Is there any way to remain strong while delivering the news that my daughter's cancer is back? Will I be able to hold back tears?

I heard Lilli and LouAnne downstairs in the basement laundry room. The window blinds sliced the late afternoon sun into a striped pattern of light on the floor at the bottom of the stairs. I paused at the laundry room door and looked at LouAnne and Lilli. "Lilli, I got a call from Dr. McLean this afternoon," I said.

"Oh, no!" LouAnne gasped, "No!" She knew what was coming next.

"He said they saw some funny looking cells in your labs from yesterday," I added. Lilli turned to LouAnne, buried her head in LouAnne's chest, and started crying.

"It's not fair," Lilli said. "Why does this have to happen again? I'm going to miss more school. And I just want to be a normal teenager!"

I explained that Dr. McLean had said there was a 75% chance that the cancer was back and that we'd have to return to clinic on Monday for another bone marrow aspirate to determine if the cancer had returned. LouAnne and Lilli hugged each other, each in tears about what they had just learned, and I joined them in a group hug. I reminded them that we had suspected that a bone marrow transplant might be required someday and that Lilli would be a good candidate for a transplant, an abstract notion to me at that time.

We walked upstairs to break the news to Amelia and Collin, and it felt a lot like the December night in 2014 when I had to tell them that their older sister had cancer. There was a good chance that the cancer was back, and we would all have our lives turned upside-down again if that were the case.

LouAnne called her parents and asked them to come back over the weekend. She said that there was no way she could go through this possible recurrence without them, and I couldn't blame her. Papa Joe and MaMaMa Janet had been so helpful during our first battle with cancer and multiple months' staying in the hospital, and we'd need their help again. They would pack up again, leaving their home, their church, their friends, Papa Joe's daylilies and chickens, and their creature comforts to live in our basement once again. I called my dad and sisters to share the news. They were all hoping and praying for a miracle, but they could sense the concern in my voice.

"LilliBug," I said, "PaPaPa Lee, Aunt Tammy, Aunt Toni, and Aunt Teri are praying for you. They're praying for a miracle." I posted an update to my Facebook page calling for all my friends and family to pray for that 25% chance that Lilli's cancer had not returned.

LouAnne and I looked at each other and said, "Let's go out to eat. Lilli, you pick the place." We couldn't just sit at home all weekend. We filled our time that weekend with eating out, shopping for things to take our minds off things, and watching Collin's Pinewood Derby car compete at the Cub Scouts' event Saturday morning. We told our scouting friends the news about Lilli's labs, and they consoled us while our sons celebrated wins and suffered losses on the track. Inside the church gym, I tuned out the chatter of young boys, the whirring of plastic wheels full of graphite powder on metal tracks, and the announcer's amplified play-by-play. While these activities happened in real time, I watched the slow-motion film of Lilli's mothering her little brother by letting him sit on her lap while she wrapped her arms around him.

That night, LouAnne and I lay in bed with the lights off. I could feel LouAnne's body shaking as she rolled over, grabbed my hand, and said, "I don't wanna lose my baby girl. I don't know what I'll do if something happens to her. It's just not fair, Travis."

"It's possible that Lilli won't make it through this. It's gonna be hard on her. I'll be here for you through all this, and we have each other, whatever happens," I said.

We rolled over to the middle of our king-size bed, held each other, and cried ourselves to sleep in the same bed that night, something we couldn't do when Lilli was first diagnosed the previous year.

89%

....

Joe and Janet arrived over the weekend with a van load of clothes and supplies to last for weeks away from home. Amelia and Collin went to school Monday morning while the rest of us drove to Winston-Salem for a day I dreaded. I felt like the leukemia was back, and I braced myself for the news. I thought that the oncologists would admit Lilli that day if the cancer had returned but let her go home if there were no cancer, and I told Amelia and Collin that they would know the results of the tests when we got home later that day, depending on whether or not Lilli were in the van with us.

We checked in to the 9th floor clinic where they prepped Lilli for the bone marrow aspirate and spinal tap before wheeling her down the hall to the elevators and down to another floor. LouAnne and I followed Lilli into the procedure room where they would put her to sleep and then take a small sample of bone marrow to be put on multiple slides. For a room with such an institutional purpose, it had one of the best views in the entire hospital. From that room, I looked out at the skyline of Winston-Salem, a beautiful sight, before being asked to leave so that they could perform the procedure. LouAnne and I kissed Lilli on the forehead, said a silent prayer, and left the room.

We walked to the waiting area and sat down. Dr. Russell came out to say that the procedure had gone well and that he had no trouble getting a sample, something that gave him some encouragement. I asked him what he thought, what his gut feelings about Lilli were. Dr. Russell said, "With AML, it's most likely a recurrence. It'll take a few hours for the lab to look at the samples, though. You all should take a break, get something to eat, and come back to the clinic after lunch for the results." He had confirmed my gut feeling and prepared me for any bad news that might come later that day.

Lilli was with the anesthesiologists when we got back to the procedure room. She took her time waking up, still with an IV in her arm and a bandage on her hip. I tried to hold her up and help her walk out of the room and down the hall, but we had to find her a wheelchair. Steering the wheelchair through the maze of corridors to the elevator, we took Lilli down to the cafeteria with Joe and Janet who had rejoined us and helped scope out a remote table and chairs.

I couldn't enjoy my lunch out of worry and anxiety, and Lilli was still too lethargic to enjoy her lunch, either. Joe, Janet, and LouAnne were also quiet and appeared distracted by their thoughts. The cafeteria had been renovated since Lilli was last inpatient in the hospital, and we decided to try some of the new offerings, even though none of us had an appetite. I was anxious to hear the lab results.

After we finished our lunches, we headed back upstairs to wait in the oncology clinic waiting room until the team shared the lab results with us. I had a knot in my stomach the entire time we were waiting. The clinic staff walked back and forth occasionally, barely making eye contact. At one point, I thought I could tell that one of the nurses had been crying.

Was she crying? Is she crying because of Lilli? Or some other patient? What if they know something they can't tell us for certain, yet? Should we start crying, too?

Dr. Russell and Kat called us into the clinic's consultation room. A dark room with dim lights that would get no brighter set a somber mood. This was the room where we would've learned about Lilli's cancer the first time around had we not come in through the emergency room late on a Friday night. We had occasionally waited in this room when waiting for Pat to draw Lilli's blood at her regular check-ups, but we had not spent much time here. As minutes passed, I started to survey the room more closely. There were shallow bookshelves all around the room with booklets on titles like "Living with Cancer, Pediatric Leukemia, Surviving Cancer," in English and other languages. I studied the various topics and grabbed a booklet on bone marrow transplants, as that's where I suspected we were heading.

When Dr. Russell and Kat sat down with me, LouAnne, Joe, Janet, and Lilli to review the bone marrow results, Dr. Russell informed us that the cancer had returned. It had come back much stronger than they had anticipated, given the way that Lilli appeared (once again I heard how Lilli could appear fine even though her cells were going haywire), and the percentage of cancerous cells was up to 89%. LouAnne gasped and grabbed my hand. What did he say? 89%? While alarm bells rang in my mind, I stayed composed enough to ask a few questions, like, "What does this mean? What kind of schedule does this put her on? What if there isn't a bone marrow match? Will her body respond to the chemotherapy as well this time as it did last time?"

There was a brief pause and a change in tone before Dr. Russell cleared his throat and responded to that last question. That pause was all I needed to know that the answer was "no." But, I listened to Dr. Russell continue by saying that there's really no way of knowing how Lilli's body would respond to the chemo. He said, "While we anticipated that her leukemia was back, we didn't expect it to be quite as robust as it is. Her bone marrow is now 89% cancer cells." While they certainly hoped that she would respond as well to the chemotherapy during this second battle, there was no way of knowing. This lack of knowing is what continually drove me crazy when it came to fighting cancer.

Why did Lilli get leukemia in the first place? Doctors don't know. Will the leukemia come back after more chemo? Don't know. Will she beat it? Don't know. What made it come back? Don't know. Will her body be able to accept cells from a donor? Don't know.

Dr. Russell said that there was something like a 99.9% chance that Lilli would have a match in the bone marrow registry. Organizations like *Be The Match* would make it easier to find those matches. What I heard, instead, was "there's a 0.1% chance that there is NO MATCH for Lilli in the bone marrow registry." I was not always such a pessimist, but I had been on the receiving end of devastating news one too many times to look on the bright side.

I asked Dr. Russell if they'd have to admit Lilli right away. He looked at Kat and then said, "No, we need to meet as a team and determine the roadmap for Lilli's next steps. We will also consult Dr. Buckley, who's agreed to be her primary oncologist. She can go back to school tomorrow for a few days and then come back on Thursday for the next step." While I had just heard devastating news, I was comforted ever so slightly by hearing that Lilli could have a few more days to hang out with friends, talk to her teachers, and plan for keeping up with school from the hospital…again. She would be walking around with cancer in her body, but the doctors seemed to trust us and her to be careful enough not to catch anything that would compromise her health. I would have to close my eyes and have blind faith in God and Lilli's community to keep her safe for a few more days.

That afternoon Amelia and Collin were happy to see their big sister in the van as we pulled into the driveway. After I had told them that Lilli would come home only if there were no cancer, they believed that she was well. I jumped out quickly to tell them the bad news that the cancer had returned and that Lilli would have to be readmitted to the hospital in a few days. Joy turned to devastation, as they discerned that our family time would be limited by hospital time once again and that their sister could die.

That afternoon, I went for a run at the park near our house. There's a 3-mile route around the park that I had been running regularly for months. On that day, I discovered that I was unable to cry and run at the same time. I ran with abandon, not worried about pace or distance, and I screamed out to the heavens when no one else was around. I started crying, and I couldn't catch my breath. I had to stop, doubled-over in pain and emotional exhaustion. After a few minutes of sobbing, I ran back to the car and headed home to spend time with my family.

The next few days went too quickly, but we made the most of the time that we had with Lilli before she went back to the hospital. We went to some of Lilli's favorite restaurants around town. We treated the kids to cake and other treats from their favorite bakery. We went shopping for things that we'd need in the hospital. Lilli got some new outfits for the hospital, too, for when she could get out of her room and wander around the hospital. And Lilli had one more Wednesday night with the church youth group. All the youth and the adult leaders surrounded Lilli in a prayer circle, laying on hands and praying over her. Her small group friends picked her up and posed for pictures that we still cherish. Dry eyes were in short supply as people reflected on the possibility that cancer could take Lilli's life.

The next afternoon I drove out to pick up Lilli after her last day at school. I had asked her counselor Ms. Denny to take some pictures of Lilli that day because it could be her last day there. Ms. Denny went above and beyond, treating Lilli and some of her close friends to a special lunch in the faculty conference room as well as taking some pictures of them for our sake. Lilli's friends came through for her, treating her like a superstar that day.

Dr. Buckley called me when I was on a winding country road to Brown Summit, on my way to pick up Lilli from school. He told me about the research he had done into the appropriate regimen for Lilli. While the oncology team had a clear roadmap that had to be followed the first time around, all bets were off after Lilli relapsed. Dr. Buckley felt certain about the chemo regimen he proposed, and he felt good about getting Lilli back into remission so that she could go for a bone marrow transplant at Duke. I asked him several what-if questions:

What if there's no match for Lilli's bone marrow?

What if there's no cord blood match for Lilli, either?

What if there's no way Lilli can have a bone marrow transplant?

I learned that there were several options for Lilli, that there were even treatments that could use my or LouAnne's cells as NK, or Natural Killer, cells to attack the cancerous cells. Dr. Buckley assured me that he would do everything he could to find the appropriate treatments for Lilli, even if it meant signing her up for trials at another hospital. I felt better after talking to Dr. Buckley even though I still had lots of fear and doubts.

The night before going back to the hospital, I walked to Lilli and Amelia's bedroom and asked Lilli, "How'd you like your own Instagram account? You'll be able to stay in touch with your friends from the hospital bed." Lilli jumped at the idea and had an account set up within minutes. And since both Lilli and Amelia had smart phones, LouAnne and I agreed that it was time for both our girls to join the social media movement with Instagram and e-mail accounts with privacy settings to keep them from stalkers. This decision paved the way for both girls to keep up with each other, their friends, and the outside world.

After breakfast the following morning, I said goodbye to Lilli before driving Amelia and Collin to school. Lilli had to ride with LouAnne and my in-laws to the hospital while I taught my classes at UNCG. I would catch up with them later that day when LouAnne and I swapped off after class. We would be back to teaching our classes on alternating days and spending those in-between days in the hospital with Lilli.

Gene Mutations

....

When Lilli began the chemotherapy treatments in March 2016 to get her back into remission, Dr. Buckley came into Lilli's room and gave us the news that Lilli's cytogenetic testing from the previous week revealed a mutation in one or more of her chromosomes that placed her in a Core Binding Factor (CBF) subtype of AML leukemia. He explained that this mutation was most likely a result of the previous chemotherapy's impact on her body and was potentially a good thing.

"You mean that her DNA now is different because of a mutation caused by the chemotherapy from last year? Her chromosomes are somehow better now that they've mutated?" I asked.

I couldn't believe what I was hearing, and tears started welling up in my eyes. While I would expect a gene mutation to be a horrible thing for anyone, the good news was that relapsed AML patients with this particular mutation were better able to survive their cancers through a particular chemotherapy regimen, called FLAG (an abbreviation for the specific chemo cocktail), combined with a bone marrow transplant. Fighting back tears of joy, I had to ask him to repeat what he said. Dr. Buckley repeated, "Yes, I've been going through some studies, and it looks like patients with this mutation have a 7-year survival rate closer to 90%, assuming the chemotherapy treatments, remission, and stem cell transplant." It sounded just as good the second time around.

He pointed me towards some research studies that had been done and the data that suggested Lilli might have a better chance of survival. While there were options for treating Lilli's recurring AML, Dr. Buckley felt confident about the FLAG treatment plus liposomal daunorubicin (DNX). It was all Greek to me, but his confidence made it easier for me to believe that Lilli could live through this. I looked at LouAnne and Lilli and asked, "Do you understand what he's saying, Lilli?" She nodded, "uh-huh," and I sensed some relief on her face. Dr. Buckley said that he'd be around if we had more questions and then left to go attend to other patients. After the awful news of Lilli's relapse, this news from him gave me hope for Lilli's future.

Curious to double-check what I heard from Dr. Buckley, I went home, logged into my campus library account, and read scholarly articles about the studies he mentioned. These studies, complete with charts and graphs and data, reiterated what he had told us: relapsed pediatric AML patients with this particular mutation and who had gone through the FLAG regimen had increased chances of survival. Lilli's original diagnosis of pediatric AML offered her somewhere between a 65% and 75% chance of surviving for five years. That percentage decreased upon her relapse to between 16% and 34%.

Really? 16%? 34%? Either of those numbers—and all the ones in between—scare the heck out of me.

I faced these percentages and tried to handle the fear, but if there were even a 1% chance of survival then I wanted Lilli to be that 1 in 100 to survive. This particular gene mutation, however, substantially increased her chances of survival. Closer to 80-90% of patients with this mutation, plus this particular FLAG-DNX chemotherapy regimen, plus a bone marrow transplant, were shown to have survived for at least 7 years.

"LouAnne, I found the research articles Buckley was talking about. D'you wanna read them?"

"No," LouAnne replied, "You know I can't look at those things."

I, too, struggled with those articles. Reading them caused me to shake nearly as much as when I first heard the word leukemia. The charts and graphs illustrated the stories of individual patients and their fates. The articles revealed that most of the patients who did not survive had died early on in their treatments for recurring AML, most within the first year of recurrence. In black and white, there was Lilli's future and other kids' pasts in data points, dots on a graph. Live through the early phases of treatments and transplant, and her chances of surviving would be pretty good. Should something serious come along early in her treatment (at the time I had no idea what those dangers would be), then that might be the end of our Lilli. While I didn't know how Lilli's body would respond to this new chemotherapy regimen, I was warier about Lilli's catching any kind of bug that could infect her body early on in her treatment. Avoid infections, and she just might live through this relapse.

After the first course of the FLAG regimen, we waited for the usual process of Lilli's immune system and bone marrow going down to nothing before coming back up. We were back to our 28-day wait-and-see schedule from the previous year. A lot was familiar to me, like sleeping in the hospital room with Lilli every other night with one eye open, listening out for specific bells and whistles from our old IV pole friend, *Beepy*, showering every morning before the doctors rounded, having a sixth sense about Lilli's health and wellness, teaching my college classes on the alternating days, and spending very little time at home in Greensboro with our other kids.

What was new and different was my own health. Lilli's teacher, Jamie, walked in one day, looked at me up and down, shook his head, and said, "I can't believe this is you. You look totally different than you did a year ago." I had lost 40 pounds by that point, and I wore new clothes from the athletics racks at TJ Maxx. The previous year, I had gotten to know the neighborhood around the hospital from our perch on the 9th floor and by driving around to fast food joints. The second time around, I surveyed the neighborhood from the sidewalks, running around at around 7 miles per hour. I managed to sneak out for a few runs on days when Lilli was feeling well, during overlapping hours with LouAnne.

After Lilli completed her chemo regimen of that round, we had a conference call with the transplant doctor, Dr. Martin from Duke University. I was at home in Greensboro that morning while

LouAnne and Lilli joined the conference call from the hospital room in Winston-Salem. "I'm sorry that we have to meet this way," Dr. Martin said. I imagined that all of his introductory conversations with families started this way. He told us about the procedures that Lilli would have to go through and the kinds of resources and support that the transplant team would offer Lilli and the rest of the family. And he said that we would come in for a preliminary meeting at Duke a month or so before Lilli would start having tests to evaluate her eligibility for transplant.

Dr. Martin explained to us that, while most people of Lilli's apparent ethnic and racial genetics would find bone marrow matches in the bone marrow registry, there was no match for Lilli. When I was growing up in the 1980s, a lack of a match would have been a death sentence. I had vague recollections of famous people going to college campuses to ask for large numbers of volunteers to be tested for potential matches. This would've been our fate, too, had it not been for advances in medicine and science.

Lilli would benefit from the medical advances in umbilical cord stem cell research. Pioneer doctors and researchers at Duke University and elsewhere had developed procedures for performing stem cell transplants using cells from umbilical cord blood and from unrelated, partially-matched donors. This, as it turned out, was our best option for Lilli, as she had no other match and no other path to survival. There have been advances in other treatment areas, like car-T cell therapy and immunotherapy; however, those treatments are for other kinds of leukemia, not Lilli's AML.

Given the limited number of cells in any given umbilical cord, Lilli would need more than one cord. Dr. Martin explained that it would likely be at least two cord blood donors for Lilli. He said that they were four-out-of-six matches. There was still was no perfect match for Lilli, but cord blood cells had been proven successful without being perfect matches. Dr. Martin explained that, while he would tell the public that he performed bone marrow transplants, it was more complicated than that and that Lilli's transplant would be a hematopoietic partially-matched stem cell transplant. There were four viable matches in their cord blood bank, and he said that they would choose the best two for Lilli's transplant.

The transplant process sounded daunting to me. I still couldn't understand how partially-matched cells from an unrelated donor's umbilical cord blood, frozen and stored shortly after birth, would know how to become bone marrow cells that totally transform and save lives. It seems like a life-saving treatment that has existed since the dawn of time, waiting to be discovered, but wasn't performed until the 1980s and 90s at a few cutting-edge hospitals like Duke.

When people would ask me about Lilli's procedures and my faith, I'd say that God had provided the life-saving cells and that scientists and doctors had been inspired to discover the processes for saving people's lives. Without the biology and the science, Lilli would have certainly died without a bone marrow HLA match anywhere on earth. And without the parents of newborns' saying "yes" to donating their babies' umbilical cords to science, Lilli wouldn't have had a source for these life-saving cells.

Following that initial phone call, I awoke to the notion that a transplant was not as automatic as I had imagined. It sounded

219

fairly straightforward: 1) go through more chemotherapy to get back into remission; 2) show little to no evidence of a residual leukemia; and 3) have a bone marrow transplant. While not easy, this sounded like a simple roadmap to follow; however, there were additional tests and steps to follow and hurdles to cross before Lilli would be approved for a transplant.

Lilli was encouraged by the call, but she was also depressed to hear that she would have to be isolated from her friends and most of her family while in the transplant unit at Duke and that she would remain in isolation for nearly a year post-transplant. She wouldn't be able to return to school until near the end of 8th grade. She was disappointed by the prospect of having to do most of 8th grade from home, being limited from going out in public.

Lilli's first month back at Brenner was a textbook case of chemo treatments. She spiked a fever a few nights after wrapping up the chemo and beginning the wait-and-see part of the month. She was able to unplug from the IV pole once her fever subsided for 48 hours, which gave her the freedom to walk around the hospital and enjoy the new Starbucks on the main lobby level. Lilli and I started going downstairs for lattes and frappucinnos every afternoon she felt up for walking out, using Starbucks gift cards that folks had given her. Lilli had to wear her huge industrial mask over her face, but she still wanted to be stylish by wearing trendy clothes and shoes when going out of the oncology unit.

One weekend during that round, Dr. McLean took a look at Lilli and said, "You should get out of here for a few hours. How would you feel about a four-hour pass?" Lilli beamed. "YES!" she exclaimed. I was shocked, but I wasn't about to argue with the doctor. He talked to the nurses on duty, and they coordinated a plan for us to escape the hospital for a while that afternoon. We couldn't go out in public, but we could take Lilli home to Greensboro to hang out at our house and spend some time in her own room. What a gift it was to be able to be normal once again. We returned that evening, and the reality of Lilli's situation hit us. After that brief jail-break, Lilli would have to remain in the hospital until her counts bottomed out and then bounced back.

One Saturday during that first month of Lilli's relapse, friends of ours from church organized a hot dog fundraiser to help with our medical bills. Lilli was in the hospital that day with LouAnne, but I was able to go to our church with Amelia, Collin, and my in-laws for some hot dogs. I couldn't believe how long the line was out the door when I got there. Not only were there people from our church in Greensboro, but there were also old friends, whom we hadn't seen in years, from many miles away. People traveled from near and far to support us financially through Lilli's relapse.

Lilli's blood counts came up, right on time, and the team discharged her to spend a few days at home. The confidence I gained from watching Lilli handle that round of chemo like a pro was tempered by a visit to the Duke Children's Health Center in Durham to meet with the bone marrow transplant team in between rounds of chemo. That visit provided a glimpse into the life-and-death world of transplants.

When we arrived at the Duke Children's Clinic we were in a whole new world. Whereas Brenner Children's Hospital operated on a few floors in an otherwise adult hospital wing, Duke had a separate children's clinic building with its own lobby, atrium, multiple clinics on multiple floors, and a gift shop. The atrium opened up to daylight, views across Erwin Road to the parking deck where we had parked, and balconies at each floor looking out into the space. We went to the 4th floor reception desk and checked in to say that we were meeting with Dr. Martin. The transplant coordinator came out and escorted us to a conference room off to the side, between the main clinic space and the infusion Valvano Day Hospital, or VDH, named after Jim Valvano, the famous NC State men's basketball coach known for his never-give-up speech while fighting cancer.

LouAnne, Lilli, and I sat down at a large conference room table across from Dr. Martin and our transplant coordinator. Dr. Martin handed us a stack of papers, including the "hurdle sheet" as I thought of it. This sheet had a list of hurdles that Lilli and her body would have to cross in order to live to the next hurdle:

Get into remission.

Have little to no evidence of blasts prior to transplant.

Go through additional chemo and radiation to prepare for transplant.

Engraft with donor cells by approximately 30 days post-transplant.

Have an ANC of at least 500 for three days straight

Have little to no evidence of old host cells following engrafting.

Wean off pain meds.

Wean off TPN.

Return "home" and to our home hospital after 100 days.

Wean off steroids and anti-rejection drugs.

Survive for 1-1/2 years without a major Graft-vs-Host incident.

Donor cells must continue to dominate, as shown in annual post-transplant check-ups.

He may as well have said, "fly to the moon," as each one of these hurdles seemed impossible to me and so far out of our control. What struck me about the whole cancer thing was how random it seemed to affect, attack, and resist. I could pray about Lilli's survival, but I couldn't do much physically to cause an ANC of 500.

When wrapping up this initial meeting we were offered a tour of the Pediatric Blood and Marrow Transplant unit, known simply as "5200" because of the suite number. To get to 5200 from the children's clinic we went back down the elevator to the main lobby level and turned to go through a long maze of hallways. We passed some diagnostic testing suites and then a fairly blank section of hallway where the artwork, watercolor paintings of the Duke Gardens, dominated before making a turn to go past an adult radiology waiting area. We made another turn where the emergency department and main hospital lobby collided.

Adult emergency room…this means folks will be coming in off the street with who-knows-what germs and bugs that could be contagious and put Lilli at risk. Avoid this intersection at all costs. Also, who designs a hospital where your most vulnerable patients with compromised immune systems have to cross circulation and breathe the same air as folks with the most unknown emergency situations?!"

We got a brief tour of the hospital cafeteria and Starbucks area so that we'd know where to find food and drink once Lilli was admitted. Then it was up to the fifth floor. We waited until there was a fairly empty elevator before we all got on board. LouAnne and I flanked Lilli like bodyguards, protecting her from strangers. Exiting the elevator, I took note of the children's-themed window marker art on the windows that looked out over the hospital courtyard and had a glimpse out to the street. From that view, I noticed that the overwhelming perspective was one looking back at a dull, grey brutalist concrete building with almost no detail. What an ugly building to have to look at in the ugliest health crisis of our lives!

Entering the 5200 suite meant walking down a long, dark hallway with a pair of nondescript doors at the end.

Certainly, this isn't the entry into a state-of-the-art medical facility. I feel like we're going into some back-of-house, hidden space like a storage room or closet or shipping and receiving center.

Once through the double doors, LouAnne, Lilli, and I entered a locker room where Dr. Martin instructed us to put on paper booties over our shoes and to wash our hands thoroughly. Some of the lockers were labeled with room numbers, and others were not. Each patient room had a locker for shoes, mainly, and we would have the option of buying new shoes limited to use on the unit or wearing booties over our shoes to prevent spreading germs from outside the unit. There was a small window in one corner that looked into a nurses' station on the other side of the airlock. There was a pass-thru next to the one door at the end of the space for sharing things, like food or medication, without having to go into the suite. The door from the vestibule into the 5200 unit was required us to wait before we were allowed to enter, preventing cross-contamination.

How sterile and institutional the unit felt compared to our experience at Brenner! Spaces were smaller. Ceilings were lower. The one dog-leg shaped hallway, narrower. The nurses' station was smaller. Efficient. Tight. Critical. 5200 was designed for efficiency, for fewer steps between procedures. Life and death were closer to one another, and inches and seconds could mean the difference between the two. There were no frills. There were sixteen patient rooms along the outside wall of the unit, each with a different pastel paint color on the walls, each with some kind of view to the outdoors. Opposite the patient rooms were the nurses' station, doctors' work room, patient and family activity room, family members' kitchen, bathroom, and laundry area.

A laundry and shower facility for parents? This is serious. We are in a finely-tuned machine for life and death, and we have the bare minimum number of family support spaces to exist with our children in the same unit without having to leave.

There was also a meditation room with a washroom and a small exam room affectionately called the *BOP*, which was described as an emergency room for patients recently discharged from the unit, as it was too risky for them to have the transplant patients go to the emergency department with the general population.

Dr. Martin showed us one of the empty patient rooms. We had been warned about how small the rooms were by the staff at Brenner who had visited patients on 5200, but I was shocked by how small it was. The room had just enough space for a bed, recliner, sofa-bed for a parent, and clear floor space for 3-4 people to stand around the bed. With five of us in the room it felt like a clown car. The room had one wall with cabinets and a sink, and it had a tiny bathroom carved out of one corner. The wall that anchored the head of the bed had just as many life-saving features and devices as the room at Brenner, just in a tighter configuration. There was a white board in one corner of the room, which I eyed and thought, "We will personalize this one, too," and a smaller white board for the details like nurse-on-call, doctor-on-call, and family emergency contacts. Where our room at Brenner had a large picture window with a view to sunsets, this patient room had a window the size of a small residential kitchen window and a view to...a mechanical yard and a blank wall of an adjacent hospital wing. What a horrible view of the outside world. If someone were to die in this room they would die with a depressing image of God's creation.

There were colorful posters at the patient room doors with words written on them like, "Joe Engrafted!" followed by ANC counts for Day 1, Day 2, and Day 3. This resonated with what Dr. Martin had just gone through with us in the conference room. "Have an ANC of at least 500 for three days straight." With as much fanfare as they made out of this hurdle, with all the hand-made posters, I felt the weight of this step. While there were many other hurdles to cross along the way, this one grabbed my attention.

Will Lilli engraft? Will she have an ANC of 500? What if she doesn't engraft? How many days post-transplant will it take for Lilli to engraft?

Outside the patient rooms were evenly-distributed nurses' touch down spaces where they could keep a closer watch on certain patients and could do some of their write-ups. Each touch down space had a monitor and computer and a task chair that were aligned such that from that point of view one nurse could look in on two patients. Each patient room had a window between the hallway and the room and a window in the door. We were going from our room at Brenner that had no view from the outside hallway and a sense of privacy to a room that felt like a fish bowl where everyone could look in on the patient. Patients and their families could control the blinds built into the windows, but the team could also open up the blinds in emergency situations or when they needed to keep a closer eye on a patient.

The visit to Duke left me shell-shocked for days. During my first month as a pediatric cancer Dad, I was ignorant to so many things that would've stressed me out more, had I known more about cancer and cancer treatments. When visiting Duke, I knew enough to be scared for my daughter's life. The bone marrow transplant process shifted from the abstract to the concrete, and each step of the process sounded like an insurmountable task for our Lilli.

After the visit to Duke I went home, changed into my running clothes, and drove to the park. The cool air hit my face as I ran up and down Herbie's Hill to the smell of 24-hour hash browns, eggs, and bacon, and thought about how close Lilli would come to death during the transplant.

Back at home, Lilli asked me to shave her head. She had gotten tired of dealing with the hair falling out and itching her in bed, and I obliged by shaving her head with my clippers. Seeing her bald again wasn't quite as emotional as it was the first time the previous year, but Lilli had never quite regrown her hair before having to go bald again. Even though she was doing school remotely, working again with Jamie at the hospital, her school friends would stop by to visit her in the hospital. Lesser friends would've made fun of a bald teenage girl, but I never heard any teasing or cruelty from Lilli's friends from church, school, or scouts.

We made the most out of the few days we had at home, and I prepared myself for the final month of chemo before going for the transplant. I was still teaching full-time at UNCG, alternating days at the hospital with LouAnne, and I was running two or three days a week to stay in shape. I was in better shape to take care of Lilli and to manage the hectic schedule of back-and-forth from one city to another, from work to home to hospital and back.

At home one day I opened my toiletries bag that I had been carrying to the hospital, and I pulled out my pill bottles. I walked into our bathroom, opened the bottles, and poured the pills in the trash. I had already stopped taking the pills months earlier, and I couldn't stand their constant reminder of my former self.

Good riddance! I'm finally in the best shape of my life, thanks to cancer.

Marrow

The beginning of Lilli's second month of chemotherapy to get into remission again coincided with the annual university symposium that I was in charge of organizing. I had been planning it for months, with the support of students and faculty from my department, and I was responsible for making sure the symposium was a success. On the first morning of the symposium Lilli and LouAnne went back to Brenner to check in and for Lilli to have another bone marrow aspirate and lumbar. While they were in the hospital, I was running this event with over 100 participants and attendees from all over North Carolina and surrounding states in the student center at the heart of my campus in Greensboro.

While at the symposium physically, I was mentally in another place, wondering about how Lilli's tests would go. I kept thinking back on Dr. Russell's pause when I asked if Lilli's body would respond to the chemo the second time around as well as it had the previous year. To me that pause meant that Dr. Russell believed there was a possibility that Lilli's body wouldn't respond to the chemo, which I've learned is code for, "the cancer's so strong in your body that the chemo won't touch it." Throughout the day I had to keep the symposium going by introducing speakers, making sure that student helpers were taking care of their responsibilities, and catching up with guests from the community and other colleges and universities. In between those tasks, however, I kept in contact with LouAnne who could report on what was going on but didn't have the lab results from that morning.

What I perceived to hang in the balance that day was Lilli's ability to go to Duke for a bone marrow transplant. If her cancer had become immune to the chemo, then she would potentially not go into remission and, as a result, not be allowed to go forward with a transplant. Not knowing how many other options there were for her, except for some hypothetical clinical trials, I was anxious to hear the results from the bone marrow aspirate and lumbar puncture.

In the middle of the afternoon—I forget which presentation was occurring at the time—I got a call from Dr. Buckley. I recognized the clinic's phone number on caller ID. I walked out of the symposium session, into the hallway, and out of the student center building into an outdoor courtyard space. There were students and faculty hanging out at the tables in the courtyard, so I stepped away from them to an open grassy area where I could talk in private. Dr. Buckley told me, "I've had a chance to look at Lilli's bone marrow under the microscope, and it looks excellent."

I had to ask him to repeat that last part. "What did you just say?"

"Lilli's bone marrow looks excellent. It has all the right kinds of cells, and they look great." He added a few more details, rattling off all kinds of blood cell types that he saw in the bone marrow. For a moment, I was totally speechless. I attempted to say something, but the words just wouldn't come out of my mouth. Dr. Buckley could tell that I was still on the phone and said, "Take your time."

"You don't know…how much…I've prayed for this news," the words finally escaped from my mouth. I could feel my chest heaving up and down as I tried to catch my breath. The phone call didn't last much longer, but I concluded that Lilli was still on track for her bone marrow transplant at Duke in a few months, and Dr. Buckley said that he'd be around the unit if we had any more questions.

What happened next was uncontrollable. I was on a large college campus, standing outside in an open grassy area with cars passing by to one side of me, the student center on the opposite side, and trees on the other sides. "AAaaaaaaahh," I screamed at the top of my lungs, spinning around and looking up at the cloudy sky. I cried out, "Thank you, thank you, thank you, God!" As soon as I caught my breath I started back towards the student center but stopped to call LouAnne first. "LouAnne, Buckley just called. It's beautiful!" I cried out. "Her bone marrow is beautiful. Dr. Buckley said it had all the right cells, and they're excellent!"

"Slow down, Travis," LouAnne said, "Are you crying? Why are you so emotional?"

"I didn't tell you this," I said, "but I was worried that Lilli's body might not've responded to the chemo and that there wouldn't be anything else they could do for her. It seems like she'll be able to have the bone marrow transplant after all."

"I guess I didn't look at it that way," LouAnne said, "but I'm glad that she's doing alright."

That afternoon I left the symposium and headed to the hospital to be with LouAnne and Lilli and to get back into the routine of our month-long hospital stays. Lilli was starting her final—we hoped—month of chemo at Brenner. While there would be additional chemotherapy and radiation at Duke, Lilli was in the home stretch of treatments in Winston-Salem.

After seeing the tiny, sterile rooms at Duke I wanted to bring some light and life to Lilli's room at Brenner one last time before we headed off to Durham. I posted a challenge to folks on our MealTrain site and my Facebook page. I asked people to help us fill Lilli's hospital room, wall-to-wall and floor-to-ceiling, with greeting cards. It didn't take much time before we had more cards than would fit on the walls. The nurses were like family members by that time, and they made sure that we got lots of medical tape to mount all the cards on the walls. Lilli got owl cards, funny cards, religious cards, hand-made cards, posters, arts and crafts, and artwork to put on her wall, and the whole family took turns putting up cards for several days. Lilli's nurses even got in on the act and brought her some trinkets and decorations, including small solar-powered owl figurines.

While the cards and the large picture window brought light into Lilli's room, the final course of chemotherapy was rough on her. There were a few days when she asked for no visitors, a sign that she was totally knocked out from the chemo. She rested most of the time, and she wrapped up her chemo on a Wednesday night. We learned from the team at Duke that Lilli would have to remain isolated from others for nearly an entire year, and Lilli was saddened by the thought that she might not see some of her friends for a year. Torn between being too tired to see anyone and wanting to see everyone, Lilli invited all her friends to see her in the hospital as soon as she bounced back from the rough chemo.

Lilli had passed one of her hurdles by having bone marrow that looked excellent, but she'd require another test to see if she would pass another hurdle. When it came to wrapping up the regimen to prepare Lilli's body for the bone marrow transplant there was a final, ultimate test done, an MRD (Minimal Residual Disease) test to seek out any remaining cancer cells. While the Brenner oncology team was capable of performing many of the labs in-house, the MRD labs were sent out to the west coast. Where the lab at Brenner was able to test blood samples that would reveal a 1 in 100 cells evidence of cancer, the west coast lab had more sophisticated diagnostics that could reveal 1 in 1,000 cells. When Lilli's cancer recurred, she had cancer in over 80 out of 100 cells; therefore, I was anxious to learn what kind of percentage of cancer cells she had after two more months of chemotherapy.

Will she be able to stay on target for a bone marrow transplant? Will there be any trace of leukemia in these 1,000 cells? What more can they do if there's still a trace of cancer? Are we going to have to change plans and go to a different hospital with risky clinical trials?

We got news from Dr. Buckley that Lilli's MRD test was negative, meaning that not only did Lilli's cancer retreat as a result of the

233

chemo but that the tests turned up no evidence of the disease. Lilli's cancer had gone from 89% to less than 0.01%. I thought that this kind of information should be shared with Dr. Martin, even though he would definitely get it online. Late one night from the living room sofa after everyone else was in bed, I texted him, "Travis Hicks, here. Lilli's Dad. I just wanted to let you know that Lilli's MRD test is negative. No residual disease."

It was in the middle of the night when I got a text from him: "Good news. See you soon at Duke."

Owl's Roost

Lilli had been discharged from Brenner in April 2016. I hoped it was for good and that we'd have a smooth transition to Duke. There were a few days between her being discharged and our moving to the Ronald McDonald House of Durham (RMHD). I had kept running through her relapse and over the two months of chemo, and I had a little time to lift my head and look at the local races. By chance, there was a race about 5 miles from our home the following morning: The Owl's Roost Rumble 3.5-mile race. With "owl" in its name it was calling out to me, and Lilli said that I should go for it. So, on a Friday afternoon, I did it. I drove to the local sporting goods store for the race bib and t-shirt pick-up. Luckily there were open slots, and I was able to register on the spot and pick up my first real race packet.

That evening I Googled, "how to put on a race bib." While I had a general idea of where to pin the bib, I learned not to put the race bib too high so as to avoid the dreaded nipple chafing. The weather was going to be beautiful, warm enough for shorts and short sleeves, and I planned out my race outfit the night before, laying it all out flat like I had seen people do on Instagram. Unlike my early running in cargo shorts and cotton shirts, my race outfit consisted of running shorts, a wicking t-shirt with a race bib pinned low, running shoes, and no-show socks.

The morning of the Owls' Roost Rumble I drove out to the park where the race would start. The runners who signed up for the half marathon got a half hour head start over those of us who were running the shorter distance. In the parking lot, I overheard some of the runners talking about the route, and I discovered a critical detail about the race. It turned out that I was running a partial trail race, and I had totally missed that detail in my rush to sign up for the race the previous evening.

What?! I've never run on a trail before. How in the world am I supposed to run a trail race?

There wasn't enough time to Google it and stress out about running on a trail before the race started. I had the chance to use a port-a-john just before heading to the group warm-up, which helped me loosen up and shake some of my jitters. I saw other runners stretching, and I copied what they did. I didn't know any better. I surveyed the other runners, trying to figure out where I might fit in the group pace-wise.

Without any pacers for such a short race I had to guess at how fast I might be compared to others and fall into place. After the national anthem and a quick countdown, we were off. I started out a little fast on the beginning downhill stretch, trying to dodge slower runners and not to block any of the faster runners. There were a few twists and turns around and down another hill towards a pond. I maintained my quick pace until I stepped off the pavement and hit a patch of grass leading to a trailhead.

Wait a second! Where does this go? This is a just a field of grass with no trail. I guess I'll just follow the arrows, other runners, and the race volunteers. It's not too bad running on grass, but wait. We're about to jump into the woods!

Then we twisted onto a narrower trail in the woods with roots, branches, rocks, dirt, logs, mud, and all kinds of hazards that I had never encountered while running through my neighborhood and around the park. The trail was wide enough for one person, which meant that we were all running single-file and that I had to keep up with the person in front of me but stay ahead of the person behind me. My pace, as long as I could keep it up, was dictated by the trail conditions and the runners around me. We ran up wooded hills and down wooded hills, across streams with large rocks, and finally reconnected with the asphalt greenway near where we split off towards the grass.

Was that it? Was that all the trail running I have to do? That wasn't too bad. Is the rest of this route paved? I sure hope it is.

Along the greenway there was enough width to pass—and to be passed by—other runners. My pace had slowed a little after the first mile. The running app on my phone let me know the pace, which was a little faster than I hoped. I didn't think I could maintain that over the remaining 2.5 miles, so I slowed down a little before the route took us back into the woods and up and down more rough trails. I grabbed a water cup before turning towards the trail.

I guess there's more trail after all. Ugh!!

Around the time I got settled into the dirt trail again, I turned around to see out of the corner of my eye two runners who looked like they were pushing 70 years old if they were a day. They had matching running shirts with some kind of running club's name on them. These guys were ringers. It was at that point that I realized that age was just a number and that old doesn't necessarily mean slow. These two old guys pranced around me like white tail deer jumping through the woods and left me in their dust, even as I thought I was holding my own.

From there until the end of the race I was just trying to hold on and not disappoint the other runners behind me, as there was no safe way to pass anyone for the final mile. My mind was tested like never before. I had to keep one eye on the person in front of me and one eye on the ground five feet in front of me so that I could dodge, dance, and tip-toe around the landscape without falling. I was running with a group of two or three other runners, and we maintained a steady, quick pace for the final stretch of the race. My reflexes kept me safe on that part of the trail.

I finally saw daylight when we emerged from the woods into a grassy clearing. I noticed there were other people, music, and cheering not far away. Then I saw the finish line, an inflatable archway with a digital strip on the ground to capture the official time from the chip on my bib. Another runner and I were neck-and-neck at that point, and I started to sprint towards the finish.

Wait a second! This person was in front of me on the trail. Is there some runners' etiquette that I should follow? I probably should slow down a little and let this person finish ahead of me.

I'm not sure that I would worry about etiquette now, but that day I slowed down a bit at the finish line and gave the other runner her own space to finish by herself and then crossed the finish line a split second later. Volunteers handed me a water bottle and put a medal around my neck.

My first real running medal!

Winded but not exhausted, I walked over to the tables where they had computers with the official times. I typed in my bib number and discovered that I finished first for my age group, men 40-49 years old. I had just run my first legitimate race with computer chip timing, and I had won my age group, which came with a small framed certificate, insulated lunch box, and water bottle prize.

I was on cloud nine. Winning the previous leukemia-themed 5k on a high school track in Statesville was a fluke for a number of reasons, but coming in first in my age group at the Owl's Roost Rumble 3.5 miler made me feel like a legitimate runner...and a trail runner, to boot.

RMHD

LouAnne, Lilli, and I checked into the Ronald McDonald House of Durham and Wake (RMHD) in the middle of the night one Sunday in late April. We worked all day to pack up our things and get to Durham earlier, but it didn't work out as planned. It turns out that it takes a while to figure out exactly what to take with you when you're moving away from home for five months, not knowing exactly when you might be able to return home. There was the 100-day magic number that was dangled out there in front of us. "At 100-days post-transplant you'll be able to return home, assuming you've been able to check off the other things from the list," Dr. Martin had said. This left our family aiming to return sometime in August of that year.

When we arrived, we checked in at the reception desk. It was a quiet, dimmed lobby and great room by the time we arrived, as most people at RMHD were in their beds by that time. The person on duty that night oriented us to the facility as she escorted us down to our room, Room 366, at the far end of the hall in the four-story wing designed and built for bone marrow transplant patients and their families. On the way to our apartment, the staffer pointed out a few of the amenities like the kitchen, dining room, classroom, and quiet room. "In the quiet room," she said, "there's a tabletop light-up angel that we plug in and leave on for 24 hours after one of our residents passes away."

God, please don't allow that angel to light up while we're here, and please, please, PLEASE don't let it be lit for Lilli.

While we were worn out from the day's packing and driving the hour from Greensboro to Durham in the dark, we still had a lot of large plastic bins to unload from the minivan, our same old 2002 silver Honda Odyssey that we bought shortly after Amelia was born. Luckily our RMHD apartment was close to one of the staircases that led out to the loading and unloading on-street parking. I had to run back and forth to bring the plastic bins to the apartment while Lilli and LouAnne made the beds and opened up enough of our bins and bags to have the bare necessities to make it through the night. Exhausted from the long hours of packing and unpacking, we all crashed in our beds late that night.

Lilli's school counselor had given our family's name to a local church that asked if there were any needy families in the school. That church blessed us with a Wal-Mart gift card with enough money on it to fill up our RMHD apartment with the things we'd need to set up our home away from home. I had gone to Wal-Mart a few days earlier to buy pots, pans, silverware, cups, sheets, pillows, towels, snacks, cleaning supplies, and drinks. I would keep using the card to add more necessities along the way, as it took a lot of supplies to maintain two homes during the time that Lilli was at Duke.

I began exploring Durham and the Duke University campus that surrounded us. The RMHD was only a few blocks from the Sarah P. Duke Gardens, one of the treasures of the Duke campus, and we took in the beauty of that garden as much as possible. Fortunately for us, Lilli was able to get out for the first few weeks of our stay in Durham, as she had to go through a whole battery of tests that kept her out-patient as long as possible. While Lilli had to wear a mask when around other people, she could enjoy the fresh air of the gardens.

By the time we moved to Durham I had been running for nearly a year. I had run a homegrown 5k and a legitimate trail run 5k, and I felt confident in that distance. I started running around the new neighborhood, too, trying to find new routes, following runners who looked like they knew where they were going. I discovered that if I started by going uphill on the main drag then I would be heading towards the Duke East Campus, which has a gravel path looping around the campus. I got to know the landmarks at one mile, two miles, and three miles back downhill towards the Ronald McDonald House. Heading the other direction took me towards downtown Durham or towards the heart of the main campus, and I ran just about every direction I could go during our stay in Durham.

Before Lilli could be cleared for transplant, she had to go through a lot of tests. We were interviewed as a family by the social worker for the transplant unit to make sure Lilli was fit socially. We took

Lilli to a neurologist's office for a test and evaluation, and she passed with flying colors. Lilli had an EKG to check her heart. Lilli's breathing and lungs were tested in a Pulmonary Function Test, or PFT. Lilli's chest was x-rayed. Lilli had a CT scan of her organs. These tests were spread out over several weeks, with some downtime between them. And while Lilli didn't have to go straight from chemo treatments at Brenner to the transplant unit, there was a sense of urgency that Lilli couldn't go for more than six weeks before going to transplant so that her old cancer cells wouldn't have time to regroup and regrow.

After several weeks of this testing, the transplant team met with us to let us know that Lilli was approved for the bone marrow transplant. They handed us a printout of a schedule for Lilli's transplant, and we finally had a date for it: May 23, 2016. This would become Lilli's Day Zero, the day she would get the cord blood cells that could save her life. The schedule mapped out the standard roadmap for treatment, including all the chemo and radiation therapies and additional drugs that would be required.

And there it is, Lilli's life and death prospects all boiled down to an Excel spreadsheet. I get it. But I can't help but wonder if a graphic designer or artist or musician could improve this way of representing my daughter's prospects of living.

Spa-spital

When our neighbor across the street heard that we were going with Lilli to Duke she said, "Oh, you're going to the spa-spital. At least you'll be in a luxurious hospital when you're going through treatment." I didn't quite understand what she meant, as the clinic and hospital spaces were okay but not as extravagant as she was describing. The 5200 tour definitely didn't expose any spa-like spaces. My experience was just the opposite of any resort, as 5200 felt hyper-clinical and sterile.

The first time LouAnne, Lilli, and I visited the adult cancer center, I finally saw what she meant. Like at the hospital campus in Winston-Salem, it seemed like all the recent money had been spent on the adult cancer wing of the campus. Approaching the Duke Cancer Center by car felt like driving up to a resort hotel. There were multiple driveways with lanes for valet parking, large expansive glass facades opening into huge lobbies, drop-off canopies that looked like they belonged in the latest issue of Architectural Record, and massive buildings that mimicked the collegiate gothic architecture of the main Duke campus. These were cathedrals to cancer. After we navigated the driveway, I realized that we should've bypassed it and gone straight to the parking deck, itself an architectural gem with gothic cathedral-like stone-framed openings and monumental scale. A lot of money had gone into building an adult cancer edifice, and a lot of people that day were heading into the parking deck that was connected via a beautifully articulated pedestrian bridge to the main structure.

After navigating our way to the bridge connection and through an older portion of the building we arrived at the main lobby. This lobby, clad in honed and polished stones and adorned by an intricate lattice-like wood slat structure hanging from an open stair, drew my eyes up past the grand piano on the entry level and towards the sky. I figured that the entire 5200 suite for pediatric blood and marrow transplants could fit in this lobby. The grandeur of the adult cancer building lobby was diametrically opposed to the tiny locker room that welcomed us into the world of stem cell transplants.

The elevator lobby was like that of a high-end hotel. We got to the radiation suite for Lilli's initial consultation and approached the receptionist's desk, like checking into a resort hotel. The waiting area where we sat following check-in was full of rich wood paneling, lush carpeting, several large format wall-mounted televisions, and a self-serve coffee and tea bar. We were called back to meet with the pediatric radiation doctor, Dr. Larrier, in a consultation and exam room. She was motherly and soft spoken and had a great rapport with Lilli. She asked if we were at Duke because of the cord blood bank program, and we said yes, that otherwise Lilli had no bone marrow match. As we talked, I looked around and saw the most exquisite exam room ever. The wood paneling on the walls would rival that of any corporate law office, and almost all the signs of healthcare implements were hidden and concealed behind crisp, modern architectural detailing.

To prepare Lilli for Total Body Irradiation (TBI) the team would have to measure her. This was a new one for us, as Lilli had never had radiation, which is mostly used for cancerous tumors and not as much for blood cancers. The radiation tech, a tall younger woman of few words who was efficient in her work, pulled out metal measuring tools that reminded me of bits and pieces from my architectural drafting kit. Some of the measuring sticks were pinned and hinged, extending out and collapsing back in to match the size of the patient. The tech measured Lilli's overall length and width and then used a flexible tape to measure Lilli's circumference in a few areas. Lastly, she pulled out a huge set of metal calipers and asked Lilli to hold her head very still. The technician proceeded to pull apart the calipers at their hinged connection and then pinched them together again, one end at Lilli's temple and the other at the back of her head, and took note of the measurements. She repeated the steps for several more measurements of Lilli's skull.

Calm on the outside, I was in shock internally at the sight of someone treating Lilli like a forensic science experiment. I had gotten used to tests like EKGs, blood pressure tests, pulse oximeters, and blood draws, but these new measuring tools reduced Lilli's humanity to static dimensions. These numbers somehow failed to acknowledge attributes like personality, love, humor, kindness, and all those traits that made Lilli special.

After the measurements and a brief consultation with Dr. Larrier, we took a peek at the radiation suite, the first time I'd ever seen one in the flesh. While I had worked on a master planning project years before for which there would be a cancer center with a state-of-the-art radiation unit and gantry, I had only an abstract understanding based on architectural drawings. Seeing the space in person was like stepping into an episode of Doctor Who (the old Doctor Who, before they got a decent special-effects budget), with its vast, dark open space with just a few objects inside, including a command module for running the radiation equipment and a slab for the patient where Lilli would lie as still as possible to be zapped by radiation. I pretended like this was all perfectly normal, but it represented the most unnatural space that Lilli would experience at Duke.

Lilli had a few radiation treatments while she was still outpatient. The first time Lilli had radiation she went with me and LouAnne, following the same ceremonial walk as for the initial consultation. We sat in the five-star hotel waiting room while on the other side of the walls there were procedures that I wouldn't wish on anyone. I pretended that this was all normal and focused on the potential good that could come from zapping our Lilli with radiation. After being called back, LouAnne and I turned over our Lilli to the team who would administer radiation. They asked Lilli what kind of music she wanted or if she had brought her own music. At least if Lilli had to go through these procedures, she could do so to the beat of her own tunes.

A little while later, Lilli emerged from the treatment room and seemed like her same old self. Whatever was at work in her body, it was happening at an invisible, granular scale. The three of us left the radiation suite, took the elevator back up to the main level, and walked the long, elegant halls back to the old children's clinic for Lilli's check-in with the transplant team. The distance between the radiation suite and the clinic was about as far as east is to west, and we slowly made our way to the waiting area of the clinic. In the small exam room, we finally reconnected with Dr. Martin. He asked about how the radiation had gone and how Lilli was feeling. "The Zofran must've helped you be able to stomach the long walk and wait."

"Zofran? Oops! We forgot to get that prescription. Lilli didn't take any Zofran (anti-nausea medication)," I said.

"Lilli, you must have a cast iron stomach, then, if you withstood that radiation and haven't been sick," replied Dr. Martin.

I jumped up and volunteered to run downstairs to the pharmacy to pick up the Zofran. I raced through the clinic, past the reception desk and the elevator lobby to the stairwell. I ran down the stairs, and as I got to the main level where the pharmacy was, LouAnne texted me, "Lilli just threw up. Forget the pills. We'll go back later. Get back upstairs to help clean up."

I was already in line and about to get the prescription. I returned to the exam room to find it already cleaned up and LouAnne and Lilli wrapping up the check-in with the team. It was too late for the medication to do any good, but we made a promise that afternoon not to forget the anti-nausea medicine before the next radiation session. Lilli would have a week's worth of radiation, mostly outpatient, with the final radiation session happening after Lilli was admitted to 5200.

By the time she had her final radiation, Lilli's body was worn down by more toxic chemo drugs and the radiation, and she was a shell of her old self by any standards. The cruelty of the transplant process was starting to sink in.

Two Cords,
Three Lives

A transplant patients' days are numbered, starting with negative numbers leading up to the day of transplant, or re-birthday, and positive numbers following the transplant on Day Zero. When Lilli was first admitted to room 15 on the 5200 unit, she was in the negative numbers and was there for radiation and chemo to get prepared for the transplant. This process brings the body close to death without dying, so that the bone marrow is like an empty vessel ready to receive the new cells. I was reminded of the butterflies in Florida and their process of turning from caterpillars into butterflies when overtaken by new, totally different kinds of cells.

During her negative numbered days, however, Lilli still had enough energy to keep going. She had learned about the STEPS Program through the child life team and was determined to get as many steps in as possible. By walking up and down the hallway on the unit and tracking her laps, she could win prizes by hitting certain milestones. Lilli was not tethered to her IV pole nearly as much as she would be after the transplant, and she walked laps like an Olympic athlete. When I was there with her in the afternoons and evenings, Lilli and I would walk laps. I worked up a sweat trying to keep up with her steps, and I was nervous that she would fall over, as fast as she walked up and down the hall.

Doctors and nurses encouraged the transplant patients to get as much exercise as possible by walking or, for some kids, riding tricycles or bikes up and down the hall. The doctors explained to us that it was critical for patients to keep exercising so that their lungs stayed healthy. Later, I would hear about several patients who suffered from fungal infections in their lungs. These infections were serious and potentially deadly; therefore, it was critical for Lilli to keep her lungs in shape by walking.

I tried to keep myself in good shape with my own exercise program to avoid backsliding. I weighed 185 pounds, down from my heaviest at 232 pounds, during those months at Duke. A few days after Lilli was admitted to 5200 when I was spending a day in Greensboro (from day to day I might find myself in Durham at the hospital, in Durham at the RMHD, or in Greensboro at home), I attempted to run a half marathon distance, 13.1 miles. I had run 9 or 10 miles once or twice, and I probably shouldn't have gone for 13.1. But I was inspired by watching Lilli go through all she had for over a year, and I decided to just go for it. I ran the distance along the greenway near home, and I did it in under two hours according to my phone's app. Later that day I checked back in to 5200 for my turn to spend the night with Lilli. "Guess what I did today, Lilli?" I said, "I ran a half marathon. Can you believe it?"

Lilli continued to receive radiation and chemo prior to transplant. Most of the chemo cocktail was familiar, but there was a new heavy hitter with an awful name that took its toll on Lilli's body.

If you're going to name a drug that plays a part in treating life-threatening illness, then here's a suggestion: Don't use the word "toxin" in the drug name!

Cytoxin was brutal on Lilli's body. It made her weak. It made her sick to her stomach. It took all the wind out of her sails. Combined with the total body irradiation sessions, the mixture of chemicals left Lilli weakened. I had seen what the other intense chemotherapy drugs had done to her over two cycles of chemo at Brenner, but this more intense regimen was unusually cruel on her body. She was pale, thin, sickly, and covered in red and pink bumps that looked like acne all over her body.

"Cytoxin is a cruel one," I told one of the nurses.

"Well, it does what we need it to do," she replied with an awkward grin.

On Day Zero, LouAnne and I were there with Lilli when she received the stem cells. I wasn't teaching that day, and LouAnne decided to take a sabbatical from work during Lilli's transplant process. We wore blue and purple in honor of the occasion, and Lilli wore her purple #LilliSTRONGER owl t-shirt. My hometown friend David, who owned a t-shirt shop, made a batch of shirts and gave them to us for another fundraiser when Lilli relapsed. We asked all our friends and family through Facebook to wear Lilli's colors or owls on their clothes to honor and encourage Lilli with their photos, which they did.

"Lilli, look at all these Facebook pictures. It looks like everybody we know is wearing their blue and purple," LouAnne said.

On the morning of Lilli's transplant the team made the rounds as usual. There were tests to make sure that Lilli wasn't feverish and to double and triple-check all her other labs to make sure that her body was ready to receive the stem cells from the umbilical cord blood. Lilli was pleased to find out that both donors were girls, not boys, even though the gender of the donor wouldn't have impacted the decision to use the cells or not on Lilli. I was just thankful that the parents decided to donate the cords, something LouAnne and I had done when Collin was born and the OBGYNs asked if we would donate the umbilical cord to science. "Why not?" we thought at the time, without knowing what would happen with the umbilical cord.

Dr. Martin told us that the donors' cells would smell like creamed corn, a result of the preservative used in storing the cells for years in a freezer or vault in a place we never saw. To my nose, however, I couldn't sense the creamed corn that I was supposed to smell. I imagined something out of a science fiction movie, but the cells came in small IGLOO coolers, the kind you'd use for a six pack of soda. The cells arrived at different times in big syringes, with labels marked in code so that the donors would be de-identified, in coolers from the Carolinas Cord Blood Bank.

The first syringe was locked into place in Lilli's IV pole and pump after LouAnne, Lilli, and I posed with the life-saving cord blood cells, and we watched the infusion drip down and through the tubes and into Lilli's central line. Drip. Drip. Drip. Drip. The rhythm of the drops was familiar, but these cells carried with them a second chance at life, not toxic chemicals. Lilli curled up in her bed, closed her eyes, and cuddled up with her blanket while the cells started to pulse into her body. This was it. This was what I had prayed for months for, for Lilli to live long enough to receive a bone marrow transplant that could potentially save her life. The process had the effect of putting Lilli to sleep, either because of the strain on her body to accept the cells or because of all the prep work of chemo and radiation that wore down her body to the point of nothing where the new cells could take root. It took 30 minutes for the first syringe of cells to drip into Lilli's body.

The second syringe came about two hours later. We failed to document the second donors' cells with the same photographic fanfare that we had with the first.

"Didn't you get a picture of that second syringe?" LouAnne asked.

"No, I thought you did."

"Oh well…those'll probably be the cells that win out, and we didn't take a picture."

Other than the gender of the donors and a general sense that the donors are most likely close to Lilli's age or younger (based on when hospitals started collecting and saving umbilical cords for medical purposes), we don't

know anything about the donors. Are they nice? Mean?
Are they short? Tall? Are they rich? Poor?

The details that define or describe people were of no matter to us. All that mattered was that someone, most likely a mother, had decided to donate the umbilical cord to research and for medical purposes and that the cord blood had been stored properly enough to be used in a life-saving transplant. In the moment of transplant, the humanity of that donor was the most important characteristic. Our daughter could possibly be saved by having some other girls' cells begin to grow in her.

Lilli was groggy during the second infusion of cells, but within a few hours of receiving her cord blood cells, Lilli was making buttons, a monthly event organized by the child life specialists in the Connection Room. Because Lilli missed out on some of the timing of the button-making we got special permission from the team for Lilli to make buttons in her room. In the nights leading up to Lilli's transplant, I was able to make a huge variety of circular photos of Lilli for her buttons and print them across the hall from Lilli's room. Lilli sat in her bed, and we pulled the overbed tray table to her so that she could make buttons in her bed. She had a list of people, close family, friends, and teachers, who would get some of her buttons. Certain doctors and nurses collected and displayed buttons from patients, similar to the restaurant flair in the *Office Space* movie, on their white coats and lanyards. Lilli had a few requests from her primary transplant team, and she obliged by making buttons for them, too.

Because of my exuberant digital printing, we had stacks of leftover circular photos of Lilli that never made it into buttons. Lilli and I decorated her room with those circles. We taped up all the leftover pictures, like bubbles all over the walls. I wanted to make the small room as personalized as possible for a 13-year-old girl, taping photos of her, her friends and family, and her old nurses from Brenner 9th floor, on her door. Lilli and I also made the white board our own by drawing a large syringe on the white board with the slogan "Grow Cells, Grow," the rallying cry for our family and all the other families in the PBMT community. Later during Lilli's stay, I drew an owl on a tree limb on the white board, and we used it to mark significant events of her transplant journey.

Lilli's transplant journey was just getting started, but within the first week or so of Lilli's being admitted to 5200, a young boy patient passed away. When the boy was still in intensive care, LouAnne met his mom in the hallway of 5200. She told us about the Facebook page dedicated to this boy's fight against AML. He was on his second bone marrow transplant, and he had suffered serious Graft-vs-Host and an infection that sent him down to the PICU. He passed away a few days later. Walking out into the hallway to go to the family kitchen to grab a snack one afternoon, I noticed the social worker walking with a sense of urgency to the meditation room across the hall from Lilli's room. Behind her were people who looked like the boy's family members, all with their heads hanging low and with red, puffy eyes. I put myself in their shoes as I thought about how I'd feel if I were faced with Lilli's death in the hospital. I never made it to that snack; instead, I turned around and went back to Lilli.

What is that family going through? They'll have to travel home to another state with their deceased son. Where would they spend the night? If I were them, would I want to sleep in Lilli's patient bed? Would I want to be as far away from that room as possible?

I pondered Lilli's future, but I tried to remain in the moment and to live each day as it came. While our previous experiences with chemo were quite predictable over 28 days, Lilli's team couldn't tell us how long it would take for her cells to engraft, or take hold in her bone marrow. They had a general idea of how Lilli's transplant process would flow, but there were a lot of variables out of their control. A few days after the transplant, Lilli started feeling the pain. The transplant doctors said that she would be in pain, then get mouth sores, mucositis, and totally lose her appetite. While there were some differences between patients, the team had a formula for post-transplant survival. When the pain hit Lilli, the team offered her a pain drip of fentanyl. This is the drug that killed Prince, and Lilli had it on demand from a pump and a handheld button to release a certain amount of this powerful opioid at a given time. The doctors were aware of the risks of addiction, however, and assured us that Lilli's dose would be limited to a small amount, no matter how many times Lilli hit the button.

In the midst of Lilli's pain, I received messages from a friend whose partner had succumbed to opioid addiction. He warned me not to allow Lilli on these strong pain meds, but I had to trust her team of experts. They assured us that they would manage Lilli's withdrawals from fentanyl when she was finally able to manage the pain without such a strong drug. In addition to the fentanyl, Lilli had between six and twelve daily and continuous IV-infused drugs to fight off infections, promote the acceptance of the transplant, prevent further damage to her internal organs, encourage the development of her new immune system, provide nutrients, and fill other needs that might crop up. I was used to seeing Lilli's IV pole with two, three, even four pumps, but the IV pole of a transplant patient was the size of a kitchen refrigerator. She had about 10-12 pumps at any given time, and each one had to be monitored frequently and regularly around the clock. The beeps, whistles, and sirens were constant from our old friend *Beepy* who somehow tracked us from Winston to Durham.

Day +9

During the first week post-transplant, Lilli continued to walk laps daily. She was allowed to be disconnected from *Beepy* for an hour every day, in the late afternoon, and we made the most of that hour. Before the hour-long disconnection on days when I was with Lilli, I would lay out an outfit of clean clothes, a towel and washcloth, and soap for her bath. Lilli bathed each day to minimize the risk of infection. I would sanitize Lilli's bathtub with antibiotic wipes in preparation. And as soon as the nurse disconnected Lilli's IV from her central line, Lilli would apply a plastic covering over her line. Then I would help her into the bathroom. During her daily baths, I was able to take note of side effects from chemo and radiation. Lilli was bald again, and her body was covered with red bumps, like the worst case of acne I'd ever seen.

After bathing, Lilli would get dressed so that she and I could walk the hall untethered to the IV pole. She had her brand-new sneakers and I had a brand-new pair of orange running shoes bought specifically for 5200. My shoes squeaked all over the unit, but I took it all in stride to keep Lilli in good health. She and I marked each lap on the unit (from one end to the other and back) with a ceremonial 360-degree high five/low five.

Despite Lilli's pain, she was able to walk every day that first week. Walking up and down the hall gave me and Lilli a glimpse into the other families of 5200 and into the life of the unit. We occasionally got to walk with one or two of the other patients. Lilli still showed tenderness and caring for younger kids on the unit when she passed them on the hall or did activities with them. She got to know some of the younger patients from walking with them and then, later, playing games with them in the Connection (activity) Room across the hall from our room.

When not walking around the unit and earning STEPS towards prizes (the team knew how to incentivize exercise to save lives), Lilli spent most of her time in bed sleeping, watching TV, occasionally doing some arts and crafts, and playing music every now and then with Trey, the music therapist. Lilli also worked with Josh, the young recent-grad hospital teacher, to keep up with her classes and to finish up the seventh grade without missing a beat. There were some complications with Lilli's end-of-grade tests, not of our making. The state of North Carolina had strict limitations on when and where students could take standardized tests, and there was no accounting for kids in Lilli's shoes. There was no way Lilli could leave the hospital, as it was a totally isolated existence until her bone marrow started working again, and there was no way the state would allow a student to take a test outside of the public school classroom. Lilli would just have to finish middle school with a few gaps in her transcript but with no holes in her knowledge.

On 5200 I attended to Lilli's needs as much as possible. In such close quarters, I could reach half of the things in our room without getting out of the recliner. I'd walk down the hall to the UV-filtered water station for fresh ice water, and I'd wash clothes on good days. After the dirty ones accumulated I'd walk across the hall to wash clothes in the parents' kitchen, laundry, and shower area. When Lilli requested it, I would sit on the bed and comfort her. And when duty called, I would grab the pan to catch Lilli's vomit. The room was tiny, and we became even closer as father and daughter in the time we spent together there.

Lilli felt the effects of the chemo, radiation, and transplant. She developed mucositis, an extreme condition affecting her mouth and throat with painful sores. She stopped eating and drinking almost immediately after the transplant and had a feeding tube for a small amount of nutrients. Lilli's main source of nutrition was TPN, or Total Parenteral Nutrition, which came in bags and was transfused via IV through her central line. Lilli's whole body itched as a result of the pain meds, and the team administered a different drug to counteract the itching effects of the pain meds. The team worked very hard to keep Lilli's body in a delicate balance while we waited for her bone marrow to respond. Lilli's bone marrow was depleted, requiring daily transfusions of blood and platelets while we waited for her new cells to engraft and begin making new blood cells. There was no textbook number to expect for her engraftment, but we were hoping and praying that the cord blood cells would kick into gear around Day +32, which was still several weeks away.

Engraftment became something that I hoped and prayed for, and I envisioned some time shortly after Day +40 or +50 when Lilli would be able to leave the unit for good. Early in our days on 5200, we got glimpses of what it might look like for Lilli to walk out of the unit and to be discharged. Within the first ten days on 5200, we collectively witnessed five different patients leave the unit to celebratory confetti parades. Each time a patient was discharged, the nurses would stop by to invite us to join them in the hallway and to celebrate with the other families in this confetti tradition.

I ran in my downtime. Running around the Duke campus in the evenings after swapping off with LouAnne allowed me to clear my head, reduce stress, and see people outside the transplant unit. I began to memorize the cracks in the sidewalk and the graffiti on the retaining walls of the railroad trestle going up the hill to East Campus. I cherished the distractions of buses, students, dog walkers, baby strollers, and squirrels that scurried across my path. After each run, I uploaded a post from my running app to my Facebook account, marking the days relative to Day Zero and celebrating life.

Day +8, 2.52 miles in Durham @ 7:52/mi…It's a great day to be alive!

Day +14

For a few days in a row Lilli had fevers that kept jumping up and down between 100 and 104. They didn't go below 100 until Day +13. Dr. Martin smiled and said, "Oh, every patient here has to have at least one fever before they get out of here. You've met that requirement now, Lilli." The transplant recovery process involved the patient's body responding to the new cells with a fever. The team was confident that the fevers were caused by early engraftment and not because of some infection.

I was at the Ronald McDonald House when LouAnne called to tell me the team's assessment of the fevers and that the team decided to begin administering some steroids that would keep the engraftment in check. LouAnne said, "The nurses told me that this means the doctors are confident about Lilli's engraftment. They wouldn't start the steroids if they weren't pretty certain." I wanted to keep my hopes in check, but I couldn't keep from jumping to the conclusion that Lilli's new cells were starting to do their jobs.

At the same time, I had trouble believing the good news that the fevers could signal engraftment of the new cells. Doubts crept in. Lilli could live to be 100, and I'd still worry that her old cancerous cells would have been hiding out for 85 years, just waiting to pounce on her. Worry-free fatherhood was a thing of the past.

What if the cell activity is from Lilli's old cells? What if Lilli's old cells are stronger than the new cells? What if the radiation and chemo didn't kill off the cancer? What if the cancer cells have attacked the cord blood stem cells?

There was life in Lilli's bone marrow, regardless of its source. Her WBC, or White Blood Count, was increasing slowly. It had been in the positive numbers for a few days, and I held out hope that Lilli was getting close to the official engraftment target of an ANC (Absolute Neutrophil Count) over 500 for at least three days running. Her ANC was still negligible, but I hoped that the WBC would drag the ANC along with it in time, as the two counts are directly related.

Lilli picked up her exercise as the pain began to subside. She was already up to 235 laps in the STEPS program, and she had a goal to win as many of the prizes as she could, starting with a custom t-shirt and Target gift cards. For every 5 laps, Lilli earned a *Step* and a small rubber footprint that she could string together. We kept her string mounted on the white board wall for all to see. Lilli developed a reputation on the unit among the nurses for her intense walking. As an avid runner by that point, I even had a hard time keeping up with Lilli's hall walking some afternoons.

264

I kept up my running on days when I was at the Ronald McDonald House and LouAnne was on the transplant unit. I had my go-to routes that I would run for 2-3 miles, and once a week I would stretch out a long run of 5-6 miles, occasionally running towards downtown Durham and back or to the hospital and back. There were a few days when I had a stomach bug and was room-bound at the Ronald McDonald House. I couldn't go to the hospital to visit LouAnne and Lilli, and I camped out in the apartment. LouAnne had to stay extra days in a row, but she was in an isolated unit that provided all the bare necessities to exist for days or weeks on end.

During the days when I couldn't go to the hospital, I shopped for supplies to replenish our RMH apartment. I also pieced together my tenure dossier. While I had taken the offer to delay my tenure the previous year, I decided not to delay it any further. I couldn't predict the future to know how Lilli would feel the following year. From the Ronald McDonald House, I sat on the couch and did most of the writing and colleting materials for my tenure dossier, which turned out to be roughly 1,000 pages of documents, representing my body of work as an assistant professor at UNC Greensboro. Getting tenure was important, particularly for the benefits of health insurance, but it wasn't a life-or-death pursuit like Lilli's transplant. I could live with myself with or without tenure, and I put together my dossier without the stress that I would've otherwise felt.

Engrafted!

Unlike when Lilli was at Brenner, we were able to access Lilli's lab results almost instantaneously. We didn't have to wait anxiously for hours for the results from the team as they rounded the following day. The nurses on 5200 would print out Lilli's labs and put them on their desk in a tray organized by room number for us to review as early as possible. On nights when Lilli stayed up late, which were most nights, the nurse assigned to her would walk the lab results down to our room. Day +19 was one of those nights. The nurse walked the printout down to room 15, and she shared the good news that Lilli's ANC was above 500 for the first time that night. With a White Blood Count of 1.2 (1,200) and an ANC or 816, Lilli was one step closer to engrafting.

The following day the primary doctor on the unit checked in to share in the positive developments, but he reminded us that it was still possible for Lilli's ANC to dip below 500. We kept our optimism in check while praying that the labs that night would still trend upwards. While I tried to focus on each moment and make the most of each hour of every day, I couldn't help but want Day +20 to evaporate so that we could jump to the labs. That night Lilli got the good news that her ANC was still on the rise. Her White Blood Count rose to 1.7 (1,700) with an ANC of 833, a second straight day over 500. One more day like this, and Lilli would get a poster announcing her engraftment. Better still, Lilli would have functioning bone marrow.

The following night was my turn again to spend the night with Lilli. Like most days on the unit, Lilli walked laps in the late afternoon after spending most of the day in bed watching TV and doing arts and crafts. I got ready for bed by grabbing my pillow off the shelf and walking down the hall for clean sheets. I stretched a sheet over the recliner and threw another sheet out for covers. I got up and turned out the lights, except for the dim light over the counter, and Lilli and I decided to watch some HGTV. After checking all the IV pumps and fluids, the nurse Kirbie drew Lilli's labs. The three of us knew the importance of those labs, and Kirbie whispered, "fingers crossed!"

Lilli and I couldn't sleep until we heard the lab results. My attention bounced back and forth from watching TV to looking at Lilli and wondering what her counts would be. About an hour after the lab draw, Kirbie walked back into the room to hand us the printout. WBC: 1.9 (1,900), ANC: 1,311. "You engrafted, Lilli!" she said. I looked over at Lilli who sat up straight in her bed. Lilli smiled from ear to ear, and I thought I could see a glint of a tear in Kirbie's eye.

After Kirbie left the room, I looked at Lilli. Lilli looked at me, raised her arms in the air, double-pumped her fists like I had never seen her do, and half screamed and half whispered, "I ENGRAFTED!" I texted LouAnne to let her know, and she FaceTimed us right away to share the moment.

"You did it, Lilli!" LouAnne said, "I'm so proud of you, and I love you. I'll call MaMaMa and Papa Joe and let them know so they can tell Amelia and Collin."

After we hung up, I started to post something to my Facebook page, but I chose the better route of asking Lilli to write something to her Instagram account that I could copy. Here's what she wrote:

"Update: Three weeks ago today, I had my Bone Marrow transplant...My immune system had basically been wiped out completely and then I entered the long period of waiting for engraftment. I had to have an ANC over 500 for 3 days straight in order to become engrafted. Day 1 of those 3 was June 11. We had heard that it could go below 500 the next day, but June 12th the ANC was over 500 again. Today the 13th of June a year and a half after I was originally diagnosed I have reached an ANC of 1,311 meaning that I have officially engrafted!!! In case any of you are confused on what an ANC is, it's basically a fancy way of saying immune system. This by no means means that I have a normal immune system. I won't for about a year, but it does mean that I am one step closer to going to the Ronald McDonald House again and having a little more freedom. I will have to stay in the hospital 1-3 more weeks just because they need to make sure I can make enough blood cells and that I can eat food and not have IV nutrition. I still have no appetite

for food and may not for the next week. Hope to be back at school and church as soon as possible."

The nurses would take time to make each patient a special poster when the patient engrafted. I had seen those colorful and personalized posters the first time we visited 5200 on our tour, and I looked forward to what the nurses would do for Lilli. Several of the crafty night shift nurses worked on Lilli's poster during their breaks. They knew Lilli well enough to put owls on the poster. They cut out a tree shape and put three owls in the tree, one for each day of engraftment with the ANC from each day written on one of three leaves they had cut out of construction paper. A large yellow sun with the words "Lilli Engrafted!" emerged from behind the tree. For as long as Lilli remained in the hospital, this poster hung from the hallway window so that other patients and family members could see. This poster was special.

Engrafting was one of the things that Dr. Martin had presented to us in the initial consultation, one of the hurdles that Lilli would have to cross in order to be released from the hospital and ultimately survive the stem cell transplant. There were more hurdles, but Lilli had jumped a major one…and faster than the average patient. I had prayed for engraftment around day +30 or +40, but Lilli engrafted on Day +19, at least a week ahead of schedule. Her day of engraftment coincided with LouAnne's and my 22nd wedding anniversary. I recall Lilli's engraftment vividly, but I can't recall doing anything special for LouAnne. Such was our life as a married couple with a transplant patient.

Within a week of Lilli's engrafting, we got a visit from Ruth, an experienced nurse whose job it was to train us on all the home healthcare tasks that LouAnne and I would have to perform after Lilli's discharge. The nurses on the unit had encouraged us to believe that seeing Ruth come into Lilli's room would be a good thing, as Ruth's training program was one of the final steps before a patient could be discharged from the unit.

Ruth showed up at Lilli's room one day with a huge binder with all kinds of instructions and information about the post-transplant experience.

This is it! Lilli must be close to being discharged. She was an early engrafter, and now she's gonna be discharged ahead of schedule, too.

Ruth came with some teaching aids to train me and LouAnne in line care and blood draws. She had a mock-up of a central line mounted to a pillow leading to a pan to catch the fluids. Even though I had some experience in flushing Lilli's central lines during those days in-between rounds of chemo at Brenner, I was a total novice at drawing blood. I couldn't stand the sight of blood prior to Lilli's cancer diagnosis, but I had to get used to massive amounts of blood over the previous year and a half. Ruth trained me on the mock-up, and she also trained me on using pumps that Lilli would have to use post-discharge. I learned how to administer the PediaSure shakes via Lilli's NG tube with an external pump, and I learned how to use the external pump for infusions of IV fluids. On alternating days, Ruth trained LouAnne on the same techniques.

How in the world am I supposed to remember all these steps and procedures?? These nurses have years of experience with all these tasks, and I'm supposed to be able to do this after a few hours' training?

After Ruth trained both me and LouAnne, we were ready to put our training into action. The nurses, upon learning that we had passed the training with Ruth, would ask me and LouAnne to do some of the basic tasks like drawing labs and flushing lines. I was nervous to do any of these tasks, but at least I had a nurse watching over my shoulder to correct me if I were to make a mistake.

Working with Ruth, we expected to take Lilli back to the Ronald McDonald House in no time. That expectation, however, would go unfulfilled for longer than anticipated. Shortly after working with Ruth and feeling like the team would discharge Lilli quickly, I noticed that Lilli was not feeling well for a day or so. My hopes for discharge were dashed when Lilli started getting worse, not better. Lilli started struggling with nausea, vomiting, pain, and lethargy. I was in denial, but the words "Graft Versus Host" kept swirling in my mind.

Graft-vs-Host

GVHD, or Graft-vs-Host Disease, was a term that struck fear
into my heart. Even before Lilli went to Duke for her transplant, a
family friend told me and LouAnne the story of a co-worker who
had died as a result of GVHD from a cord blood transplant. This
friend of a friend had opted for an optional bone marrow
transplant to escape a chronic case of leukemia, and this person
had died from the side effects that could attack any transplant
patient, including our Lilli. I couldn't get that story out of my mind
throughout Lilli's transplant journey.

Lilli's body was the host, and the new umbilical cord cells were the
graft. While the new cells were mostly a match for Lilli, 4 out of 6
HLA markers, they were still different enough to fight against
Lilli's cells and her body. Even when the transplant team said that
"a little GVH is a good thing, because you also will get the GVL or
Graft Vs. Leukemia effect," I still prayed that Lilli would not get

Chronic Graft Vs. Host Disease, as it could kill a patient who suffered from it badly enough, or if she did get GVH that it would be a mild enough case that she could survive it.

Lilli started to break out in a rash around the time of her engraftment, and the team felt certain that it was a sign of GVH of the skin, a good thing apparently because skin GVH is easier to fight with steroid cream. For several nights, we had to slather Lilli's exposed skin with a thick layer of a greasy steroid cream and then wrap her up like a burrito in a sacrificial sheet, not her nice sheets that we had bought to make her room special. It had been a week since Lilli had gotten over her skin GVH, and this new development in her condition was much scarier.

Lilli was sick to her stomach for a few days, around the time that the team started talking about discharging her and letting us go back to the Ronald McDonald House. I prayed that she would not have a bad case of Graft-vs-Host, as this was one of the hurdles that was presented to her. I continued to watch her get sick to her stomach, something that was not common for her. The lead doctor one day said, "we should probably rule out GVH," after Lilli's symptoms worsened. One night Lilli called for her bucket, the pan kept beside the bed or even closer when Lilli could tell she was going to throw up. She proceeded to vomit something the likes of which I had never seen before nor since. It was dark green, practically black, and seemed to come from deep down inside her. I was scared, worried that she might have a scary infection or, even worse, a bad case of GVH.

Within a few days, Lilli was scheduled for an endoscopy to test for the presence of GVH in her upper GI tract. That morning I awoke to a wheelchair and escort at the door to take Lilli down to the surgery suite. LouAnne was trying to get to the hospital in time for the procedure, but the wheelchair beat her to the room. I walked down with Lilli and the escort, continuing to worry about Lilli and what was going on inside her GI tract. This was the first time Lilli was allowed to leave the unit, but there was no confetti parade for an endoscopy. I prayed that we would not encounter any sick people between 5200 and surgery.

The doctor who checked in Lilli to surgery and the GI specialist discussed the process of the endoscopy with me and Lilli and told us that they would give us a preliminary report following the procedure. After they knocked out Lilli with anesthesia and wheeled her back for surgery, I left the prep room with Lilli's bag of possessions, some clothes, sneakers, an iPad, and headphones, and headed to the waiting room where LouAnne would meet me after driving over from the RMHD. We sat down with the other families who were there with their children and grandchildren, and I tried to remain positive amidst the threat of one of the scariest conditions I could imagine at that time.

If the donor's cells are too weak and not winning the fight, then that could mean that Lilli's cancer could return. If the donor's cells are so strong that they affected Lilli's organs, then that could mean organ failure.

I prayed for the delicate balance required in order for Lilli's new cells and old cells to find a harmonious balance in which the donors' cells would take over and kill all the cancer.

One of the moms from 5200 was also there in the waiting room. I didn't expect to see her there. Her daughter, a little younger than

Lilli, had been right there in 5200, hanging out in the activity room and walking laps around the unit with Lilli. Now both girls were in surgery at the same time. This mom talked more to LouAnne than to me, as LouAnne is really good at making friends in the hospital and at sharing stories with the other moms and dads. I'm more introverted and generally kept to myself around the other parents and family members. I overheard this other mom describing how her daughter's kidneys had shut down and how it looked like there was nothing else the doctors could do for her. I couldn't imagine hearing that news, but I also thought "what if something like that were to happen to us?"

A few days later we heard that this family was checking out of the hospital and heading back home to another state, as the team on 5200 suggested that they had done all they could for their daughter and that the family should go home, call their families, and get their affairs in order. LouAnne continued to keep up with this other girl and her family, and she was one of the miracles we witnessed, living through this dire prognosis and surviving despite all the odds against her.

After Lilli emerged from the endoscopy, LouAnne and I were called into a consultation area. We entered from the waiting room side of the room, and the endoscopy specialist entered from the staff side. She shared with us some photographs of the inner lining of Lilli's upper GI tract and some initial gut reactions—no pun intended—to the results. She said that visually the GI tract looked okay (not an enthusiastic reaction, I thought) but that the biopsy would tell the accurate story about GVH in a day or two. After this, LouAnne and I were called back to the recovery area where they brought Lilli out of her sleep and checked her vitals before sending her back up to 5200.

Several days later, we found out from the transplant team when they rounded that Lilli in fact had a case of GVH. The lead doctor who was on that day emphasized the positive of this result: "While she does have a case of Graft-vs-Host in her upper GI tract, we know that she will also benefit from the GVL, or Graft-vs-Leukemia effect." I thought about how much of a balance this whole transplant regimen was. You want to have a little GVH, but not too much. You need to use some anti-rejection medications to keep the new cells at bay, but using too high a dose of those meds could ruin the transplant's success. You need some steroids for some of the same purposes, but too many steroids and your blood sugar goes through the roof. I tried to hang on to the positives as the doctor presented them, too, but I couldn't help but worry about a bad case of GVH, as this was one of the hurdles in Lilli's Olympic-sized plan. Lilli had not yet succeeded in jumping that hurdle.

In spite of this case of Graft Vs. Host, Lilli continued walking laps except for one day when she felt awful. That was the same day when she asked me to sit on the bed beside her, something that she rarely did.

"Daddy, can you come sit with me?" she begged, "I don't feel well."

She was itchy and tired and loved it when I scratched and rubbed her back while she sat in my lap and cuddled with me. She reminded me of that same little girl who sat on my lap in church until she was in sixth grade and who liked to hug and love on people.

Feeling better the following day, Lilli walked her 500th lap on the unit and earned her 100th "foot," joining the 5200 Century Club for having over 100 rubber feet strung together. For this achievement, Lilli had her name published in the transplant unit's monthly newsletter and her picture mounted on a poster in the hallway for all to see. Despite the GVH diagnosis, we continued to follow the treatment road map and pray for the best.

Day +34

....

The team felt good enough about Lilli's progress and the status of her immune system to give her a two-hour pass from the transplant unit around Day +34. LouAnne and I were both there with Lilli so that we could hear the instructions for taking her out of the unit. We couldn't go far away from the unit, and we had to be back in two hours so that Lilli could stay on track with her IV meds. In her weakened state, we borrowed a wheelchair from the hospital to wheel her out of the unit, down the elevator, out the main lobby, across Erwin Road to the parking deck, and then on to the Ronald McDonald House. This was a test run for our family. If we could manage to keep Lilli healthy over the course of two hours, then we'd be rewarded with another pass and another and another until Lilli was discharged.

Lilli had not been out of the hospital in five weeks. She had not even left the transplant unit in that amount of time except to have

278

an endoscopy. She was ecstatic to be outside on a beautiful summer evening, and I was elated yet nervous to escort her outside the hospital and down the road to the Ronald McDonald House.

Lilli turned out to be an early engrafter, and aside from GVH, she had dodged infections and viruses, life-and-death emergencies, and trips to the intensive care unit for the time she was on the 5200 unit. To see her outside the hospital while having a relatively easy transplant process to that point, I was grateful for her life. I was also nervous that I would break Lilli or do something to expose her to an infectious disease that could kill her. With limited time away from the hospital, Lilli chose to hang out in our apartment, not doing much but watching TV with the family in her home away from the hospital. We lingered for a while outside the apartment on our way back to the hospital, not wanting to miss out on a second of freedom.

The following morning, the team of doctors rounded and had an important announcement to share with us. Again, LouAnne and I were both there, something that rarely happened except in the evenings when we swapped places. We both stood up in the tight space around Lilli's bed because there were five adults plus Lilli in a tiny room. Dr. P., the lead doctor on 5200 that week, asked one of the fellows to share the news with us. She calmly and quietly said something to the effect that the lab results showed greater than 98% of Lilli's cells were from Donor #2. Even though I was standing near the doctors, I had to ask her to repeat what she said.

"The results show no trace of Lilli's old cells," she repeated.

Is this what I think it is? Did she just say what I think I heard?

Dr. P. repeated the news, in a loud and clear voice, "In medical terms, we would consider Lilli's transplant a success. The donors' cells have been winning against Lilli's old cells." He went on to hand us some paperwork with the results from tests referred to as chimerism tests. These tests revealed the DNA results from three different fractions of blood circulating in Lilli's body. My wish from Day Zero was that Lilli's old cells would lose in an epic microscopic battle with the umbilical cords' stem cells. The printout of the lab results illustrated how strong the new cells were against Lilli's old cells. Over 98% of the cells in each of the three fractions were from Donor #2, the second syringe transfused into Lilli's body on Day Zero. Why not 100%? The lab apparently hedges on its results, recognizing that a blood sample can't accurately represent all the blood cells in one's body. According to Dr. P., we could think of the >98% the same as we would 100%, as the tests showed no detectable trace of Lilli's old blood cell's DNA.

I looked at LouAnne, and she started tearing up at the news about Lilli's successful transplant. I, too, was overwhelmed by the news. This was the news that I had hoped for but feared we wouldn't hear, as we were reminded from time to time that 15% of the transplants are not successful. Lilli had already been on the losing end of percentages as a cancer patient, but at least for the moment she was winning the battle against cancer with the help of doctors, nurses, medicine, scientists, researchers, and someone's little baby's umbilical cord blood cells. At some point a mother and father had decided to donate their newborn's umbilical cord to science, and that decision had given Lilli a longer life.

While their sister was going through this life-saving process, Amelia and Collin were amazing in their own strength and support of their big sister. They visited the transplant unit when possible, participating in family-oriented activities. They worked on some arts and crafts projects, like making little birds out of feathers and clay and pipe cleaners. They kept Lilli in good spirits by simply hanging out and watching TV or playing games with her on 5200. They did all this while continuing to be kids and to do kid things like go to school. Amelia's fifth grade celebration occurred during Lilli's stay on 5200, and LouAnne and I recruited Tammy to stay with Lilli while the two of us were able to go to the celebration. Collin wrapped up second grade, too, during Lilli's time at Duke.

LouAnne and I tried to spend as much time as possible with our other two kids, but one of us had to be with Lilli at all times while she was inpatient. I sensed that jealousy could creep in as Amelia and Collin watched their big sister get all the attention, so I put out a request for all our followers on Facebook and MealTrain. I challenged folks to mail cards of encouragement to Amelia and Collin, and our community once again came through. The mailbox at the Ronald McDonald House was stuffed with cards to our family, mostly to Amelia and Collin, and some people were kind enough to send small gifts and gift cards.

After school ended for all three kids, Amelia and Collin could finally live in Durham with us at the Ronald McDonald House. We still had help from Tammy, Joe, and Janet to keep up our home in Greensboro, but we could begin laying the groundwork for our family of five to be together again in the RMH apartment.

Confetti

Aside from the 100-day post-transplant mark, there were other milestones in the transplant process that we eyed from our first days in 5200. One of those milestones that punctuated Lilli's hurdles was a confetti party, a tradition in which patients and patients' families would be showered with confetti as the entire unit celebrated their being released from 5200 out into the world. In our case that release was out to our room in the Ronald McDonald House on July 5, 2016, just over six weeks post-transplant. The previous day was the 4th of July when Amelia, Collin, and Lilli joined in special activities, games, and a parade hosted by the family life staff. The unit was awash in red, white, and blue.

While Lilli's room on 5200 was tiny compared to the rooms she had at Brenner, we still had managed to accumulate a lot of stuff during the six weeks we were there. Believing that Lilli was bound to be released the next day, I started packing up our stuff the night before, after we returned from Lilli's 2-hour pass. I was still packing the following morning when the team rounded to check on Lilli and make sure she was ready to be discharged. Lilli's temperature that morning was borderline, almost to 100, but on the second check it had dropped enough for her to be given the all-clear. There were plenty of discharge procedures for us to follow, however, and it took several more hours before we got our confetti parade.

The music therapist, Trey, played guitar and sang, "There she goes…" as we headed down the hall toward the locker room where we would perform our best Mister Rogers impressions and change our shoes before going out into the world. Families came out of their rooms and cheered for Lilli, throwing confetti at all of us. It was a family affair for us, as Amelia and Collin came to join in their sister's celebration with me and LouAnne. We all had colorful paper confetti in our clothes, bags, and cars for several months after that celebration.

It wasn't too long before Ruth, the discharge nurse, paid us a visit at the Ronald McDonald House. She trained us on the various tasks we would have to do for Lilli once we were on our own. I couldn't believe the scope of daily nursing and home care that we would have to perform on our own daughter. Why would they trust a parent to perform medical tasks that take nurses years to master? I could understand the love and caring that I would show Lilli, but I had never drawn blood before the few times on 5200 under the watchful eyes of trained nurses. And now they were asking me to draw her blood every single morning for weeks after she had been discharged.

The Pediatric Blood and Marrow Transplant unit sent us home with a few things to help us with the regimen that we would need to follow. In addition to Ruth's help, we had a white binder with all kinds of information printed out for our use. It didn't cover every situation we could find ourselves in, but it covered the standard protocols and had emergency phone numbers for the unit and the 24-hour on-call team. We also got a small black insulated lunch box to use for our clinic visits. The pharmacy sent over a mobile IV stand on wheels and a backpack to house all the pumps and IV bags that Lilli would need over the days and weeks to follow. We also had syringes, vials, saline, heparin flushes, IV pumps, and enough batteries to power a small city. And the pharmacy would keep sending boxes of batteries to us every day. There was no way Lilli's pumps would go dead.

Most importantly, the team made sure that LouAnne, Lilli, and I each had one or more pairs of plastic clamps for Lilli's central line. Each one of the three lumens could spring a leak or burst, leaving Lilli to bleed out if not for one of these life-saving clamps that looked like a small pair of scissors without the metal knife edge. We each had to practice using clamps before they would let Lilli out on passes, and we asked the nurses for as many extras as they could get away with giving us. I kept one in my computer bag for a long time, and I kept a second one in the sun visor of my car. Lilli kept one each in her lunch box, backpack, and computer bag. LouAnne kept one in her purse and another one in her minivan. We were prepared for a burst line.

LouAnne and I were in charge of filling Lilli's NG feeding tube pump plus another pump with chilled TPN nutrition bags that would be delivered to the RMH every afternoon. We would have

284

to connect the TPN pump every night, several hours before going to bed, and hang the portable NG feeding tube pump on an IV pole that Lilli could wheel around the small apartment by herself in the middle of the night. We would have to monitor this pump throughout the night and disconnect the tubes the following morning when the alarm would start going off. After disconnecting the nutrition from Lilli's feeding tube, I would switch modes from feeding to medicating. The medications involved around 20 different pills and capsules that Lilli would have to take several times a day. We kept a spreadsheet of all the pills and checked them off one by one before taking them to Lilli who would still be lying in her bed. LouAnne and I worked together now that we were back in the same place after being separated for weeks.

Lastly, each morning we were responsible for drawing Lilli's blood from one of her central lines, of which she had three, labeling the three vials of blood, and then driving the samples over to the Duke Children's Health Center where I'd run them upstairs and deposit them at the lab drop-off basket near the nurses' station. After a few days of this, Lilli expressed a preference that I be the parent to draw her blood. I obliged, even on mornings when I had to leave Durham to teach my summer studio at UNCG. We were also responsible for changing the caps on those central lines as part of the routine procedures. Again, each one of those lines was a direct conduit from the outside world to Lilli's heart. LouAnne and I had a huge responsibility.

I am pretty squeamish around blood, yet here I am having to draw her blood each and every morning, something that had been done by her nurses for months. What did I know about being a nurse? Surely the brief training sessions I received couldn't prepare me for all possible situations.

For each blood draw, we all had to maintain a sterile environment, wiping down surfaces with alcohol wipes, wiping anything that would touch Lilli's lines with alcohol wipes, wearing face masks over our mouths, and wearing sterile gloves. The risk in all this was that we would accidentally forget to sterilize something or make some mistake in executing these nursing tasks, putting Lilli in danger of some kind of infection as a result of our mistakes. I took ten minutes to prepare all the syringes, vials, and other tools and lay them all out on the cafeteria tray that Ruth had loaned us when Lilli was discharged. I prepared the tray on the small kitchen counter before carrying the tray into the bedroom where Lilli had one of the two full-sized beds to herself.

One morning my fears about line care came true. I was going through all the steps in the process to draw Lilli's blood and to change the caps on her lines. I would first draw the blood and then change the caps. The blood draw procedure didn't require that we wear masks, but a cap change did require us to wear masks. Without thinking, when I finished drawing the blood into the syringe and went to push the heparin flush into the line I inadvertently removed the cap from Lilli's central line along with the syringe, leaving one of her lines exposed to the germs from our breath. I locked eyes with Lilli with a look of horror. The line to her heart was essentially open without a cap and without a cap ready to attach.

Oh no, Lilli! What did I just do? I wasn't thinking!!

We had to act quickly. As fast as I could, I prepared a fresh cap on the end of a syringe of heparin and screwed it onto the end of the open line while Lilli scrambled to grab a mask and cover her face. I yelled to LouAnne, who was sleeping in the other bed, to get out of the room since we only had two masks. I covered my nose and mouth with a mask as soon as I had the cap on the line. Luckily Lilli had closed the clamp on that line before I unscrewed the cap, so the only exposed section of line was from the end of the line up to the clamp. After I secured the new cap and syringe to the line, Lilli and I looked at each other, thinking the same thing.

Calmly, Lilli said, "Don't open the clamp, and don't push anything from the syringe into the line."

"What should we do, LouAnne?"

"We should take her to the clinic."

I called the clinic, described our mistake to the team on call that morning, and they were very calm. They instructed me to leave everything as it was, including the syringe hanging off the line, and to come straight to the clinic to draw blood cultures and to flush out the lines. The nurse ran an IV antibiotic drip, in case there was any infection caused by my mistake. The team wasn't too concerned, as we had made certain not to unclamp the line, but that didn't keep me from worrying.

I worried about what I could've done to Lilli for days after that. The closest we had come to losing her was the previous year when she had sepsis and a blood infection, essentially the same thing that could come from allowing the central line to become infected by something in the air, in the syringes, or in the process of handling those draws and pushes in and out of her lines.

This is exactly why they shouldn't let parents who are not professional medical clinicians do these kinds of procedures on their kids. What if I've put the wheels in motion for Lilli to get some horrible infection that kills her? I'll never forgive myself.

We kept a close eye on Lilli for several days after that escapade. And we managed to survive that one unscathed, as Lilli didn't develop any infections resulting from my miscue. As a teenager, Lilli was able to participate in all those home health procedures and contribute to problem-solving, like she did that day with her quick thinking. She helped me recall, step-by-step, what we were instructed to do in different scenarios. While there wasn't a textbook scenario for the mistake that I had made, we had received plenty of instructions on maintaining a sterile environment and what to do in case of certain emergencies. I prayed that we'd not have to use our wits again in such an emergency.

Day +54

Lilli "escaped" from 5200 around Day +41. **For the first six days** out of the hospital she had daily appointments with the bone marrow team in the fourth floor outpatient clinic. LouAnne and I had become full-time nurses, even though I was teaching a summer studio at UNC Greensboro an hour away. On Tuesdays and Thursdays, I would leave Durham, assuming Lilli was doing well, and drive to Greensboro, returning to the Ronald McDonald House each evening in time for our evening routine.

By Day +54, Lilli was doing well enough to go from clinic appointments 7 days a week to clinic appointments on Mondays, Wednesdays, and Fridays. On clinic days, I would drive the blood samples over to the clinic as early as possible. Some mornings I'd swing by George's Coffee near the hospital and grab a latté before heading back to the Ronald McDonald House. After a quick breakfast, Lilli, LouAnne, and I would pack up Lilli's lunch box with snacks and meds along with Lilli's backpack full of IV fluids and pumps connected to her central line. We'd drive over to the parking deck across from the clinic, walk across the street to the clinic, go up to the 4th floor, and check in. The clinic waiting area had a designated space for all the transplant patients, a bullpen separated by partial-height partitions, and we'd wait there until they called Lilli.

On Mondays, Lilli would get infusions of IVIG, a drug to help boost her immune system, which would mean a longer day in the clinic. We would spend between one and five hours in the clinic, depending on Lilli's progress towards recovery. Sometimes Lilli would need an extra dose of some vitamin or mineral to balance the effects of the transplant and the dozens of medications she was taking. Lilli had graduated from Neupogen, a drug that boosted her white blood count. Most patients were still taking Neupogen at this point, but Lilli had been able to discontinue this drug by the time she was discharged from 5200. She was the model patient for the number of drugs from which she had weaned. Lilli had also gone a long time without blood or platelet transfusions. She hadn't needed those transfusions since she was inpatient. The signs of properly functioning bone marrow were there when we looked for them. It was hard, however, to look beyond the tasks at hand.

There were the clinic days when Lilli would get a dose of Pentamidine, a drug to help prevent against pneumonia. During those treatments, which began when she was still inpatient in 5200, Lilli would be enclosed in a one-person-sized plastic phone booth looking enclosure. This negative pressure booth would be for Lilli to sit while breathing through an inhaler tube and hose connected to the vaporized medication. These treatments were administered in fish bowl-like glass-front exam rooms in the Valvano Day Hospital. While I could be in the room with Lilli during these treatments, I had to wear a mask on my face so as not to breathe in the drugs. There continued to be a lot of attention given to strengthening Lilli's lungs and preventing pneumonia and other lung infections.

On shorter clinic days, we could be in and out of the clinic in an hour or two. On days when the lab was humming along and I was able to get the blood samples there early, Lilli's blood counts would be ready as soon as we showed up for clinic. If Lilli's labs were stable, then we'd have a short visit. We would have a few hours between leaving clinic and preparing Lilli's meds and pumps for the evening cycle. I encouraged Lilli to get out and walk as much as possible, and on weekends the whole family would be there to hang out with Lilli.

Amelia and Collin enjoyed hanging out with Lilli in Durham. We spent a lot of afternoons and evenings walking around the neighborhood near the Ronald McDonald House or at the Sarah P. Duke Gardens. Pokémon Go had just launched, and we ran into a lot more people in the gardens after Lilli's transplant than we ever did pre-Pokémon. Collin began playing the game, and he was able to persuade Lilli to walk around the gardens, getting in her steps outdoors instead of in the transplant unit.

In the evenings, LouAnne and I would start again. Before we sat down to eat dinner, I would start preparing Lilli's overnight pumps, meds, and dietary supplements. The pump for Lilli's lipids had been discontinued, which left us with just the three pumps for TPN, cyclosporine, and PediaSure. Those pumps required my clearing off the kitchen counter, laying out the refrigerated IV bags, which arrived by courier each afternoon from the hospital pharmacy, connecting everything in the backpack, priming the pumps, and then having them ready to connect to Lilli's central line. This prep time took about 45 to 60 minutes each evening.

Dinner was a struggle for Lilli, not for us. We had to squeeze in the time to cook and eat or walk down to the Ronald McDonald House kitchen to grab dinner, but Lilli still had a problem with her appetite. It had been well over a month since she had eaten much of anything, but I kept pushing all kinds of food in her direction. She slowly began eating again, in small portions, things like pasta, eggs, okra, cabbage, purple hull peas, and applesauce.

The Ronald McDonald House was always full of fresh food; however, Lilli rarely partook of those meals that were provided by outside groups. The rest of the family ate in the RMH dining hall or took the food back to our apartment. One day I was humbled to be served a meal prepared by local architects and engineers, including people with whom I had worked. I was on the receiving end that day, and I looked forward to times when I could serve others in similar ways.

Day +55 was a Sunday, and it was the date for *LilliPALOOZA*, a fundraiser concert thrown by Mary, the mother of one of Lilli's close friends from school. Mary, her husband, Mark, and their neighbors and friends had hosted several backyard concerts and fundraisers at their home, and Mary offered to do the same for Lilli and our family. We just needed to assemble some talent in addition to the house band from the neighborhood. Lilli's friends asked around and got a volunteer from Lilli's grade to play electric guitar and sing. I volunteered myself on Irish bagpipes and low whistle and Amelia on banjo. We had originally planned on having Amelia's teacher on guitar, but he had a gig that evening and couldn't make it.

We then secured the main attraction for the evening, Chad Eby on saxophone with his jazz band plus his teenage son. Chad, a neighbor of ours and a member of our middle school carpool, volunteered his time that evening, but he went beyond the call for at least a month leading up to the event. Chad agreed to donate the funds from all of his CD sales during that time, and he also took donations for our family at each of his concerts or gigs leading up to *LilliPALOOZA*. What a gift.

The evening of the backyard concert was beautiful. As the mature hardwood trees shaded our gathering, people came with their folding chairs, donations, and appetites for the meal that had been prepared. A homemade wooden stage anchored the corner of their backyard in a historic neighborhood full of 1930s and 40s bungalows and craftsman homes. The yard was a hive of activity, packed with Lilli's friends, teachers, neighbors, church family, and strangers. If they came for good music, they found it. If they came for food and good company, they found it. People came for all kinds of reasons, and I was thankful for the generosity and kindness of friends and strangers.

LouAnne stayed with Lilli and Collin while I attended the concert with Amelia, my sister, Tammy, and my niece, Sidney. From a laptop computer Lilli's friends skyped her in to the concert. We took a moment near the beginning of the concert to recognize Lilli. Everyone waved and cheered her on. I spoke for a few minutes about Lilli's fight against leukemia and the bone marrow transplant that had, to that point, saved her life. From the Ronald McDonald House, Lilli, Collin, and LouAnne watched the concert.

The musicians did not disappoint. From jazz to pop to rock to folk music, there was a wide range of music, and it flowed from the heart. People sang along. People danced. They ate and drank and had a great time. People from our church came to support us. Neighbors and friends came. People passed the hat. Mary kept up with the donations throughout the evening, and she presented me with an envelope with thousands of dollars at the end of the evening. Chad also handed me an envelope full of cash, thousands of dollars from his concerts and CDs. I couldn't believe the generosity of our community that night. People sacrificed from their own budgets to help us with our budget. My faith in humanity had yet again been reaffirmed by the actions of people in Greensboro, North Carolina.

BK + the BOP

At nine weeks post-transplant, Lilli had a rough week following the high notes of the *LilliPALOOZA* concert. She dealt with several hiccups, including trouble with her feeding tube and a bout with a virus. Both of these issues caused us to make unscheduled, unplanned trips to the hospital in the middle of the night and the clinic on a weekend.

The Tuesday after the concert Lilli pointed out some blood in her urine, a shock to me. LouAnne wasn't quite as scared as I was because she had talked to some of the parents of post-transplant patients and heard about a virus that caused such symptoms. LouAnne monitored Lilli throughout the day while I taught my studio in Greensboro. When I got back to Durham, LouAnne told me that we should call the transplant team and ask what to do. The after-hours nurse advised us to come back in to 5200 and report to

295

the *BOP*, the makeshift emergency exam room on the unit, just across the hall from Lilli's old room.

We checked in late that Tuesday night to the *BOP*, and it wasn't long before the nurses took some urine and blood samples for the lab. They were fairly certain that Lilli had the BK virus, the same virus LouAnne had heard about, but they wanted to see the lab results before letting us go home. I kept my hopes up that we wouldn't have to stay very long in the *BOP*, because it was a tiny space that must've been a closet converted into an exam room out of necessity. Lilli and other post-transplant patients would not be safe going into a general emergency department with all kinds of bugs. The *BOP* did the trick for us that night.

For three of us to occupy that room meant that we were on top of each other and fighting for space. In the midst of all the stress I felt, I still had to manage Lilli's nightly PediaSure nutrition and the pump that went with it. Lilli was struggling to take all the tube feeding, and I found some comfort in having a nurse to provide us her expert opinion about the feeding tube. She said that we were doing everything by the book but couldn't tell us exactly why Lilli struggled with the tube. She suggested running the pump at a slower rate and using less PediaSure.

When Lilli got to the BOP, she had a clean-looking urine sample. "Wouldn't you know it. When we need her to have blood in her urine for an accurate lab result, it looks clear," I said. After a few hours of monitoring and running the labs, the team came back with a positive result for the BK virus. While this news wasn't nothing, the BK virus was not nearly as scary as Graft-vs-Host. The team prescribed additional fluids, which they began administering that night, to help flush out the virus. The team discharged Lilli at around 2:00 in the morning.

I felt relieved to walk out of the hospital within a few hours of arriving. Walking out of the lobby, LouAnne, Lilli, and I bumped into Dr. McAlister, one of the fellows who was on the unit in the evenings, particularly during the time when Lilli had skin GVH and required the burrito wrap with steroid cream and a sacrificial sheet.

"We just *BOP*ped in and *BOP*ped out," I said.

Dr. McAlister was all smiles. "That's what I like to hear," she replied, with a bounce in her step.

We left the lobby in the cool night air to a clear sky. I could see the stars as I looked up and said a quick prayer of thanks that we had some of our freedom back.

Lilli's feeding tube still nagged her. When Lilli was discharged from 5200 she still had an NG feeding tube. She had volunteered for one, as it was one of the things that Dr. Martin said could help her escape the unit more quickly. The other thing was walking the unit and getting in her steps, which Lilli did with flying colors. The feeding tube, however, was something that was a struggle from the beginning. When Lilli had been at Brenner she had not needed a feeding tube. We were told that chemo would lower her appetite, but the Brenner team supported giving Lilli appetite-boosting medications to keep up her weight. Lilli took this medication, and she maintained her weight during her treatments before going to Duke.

The team at Duke, however, did not believe in giving Lilli any kind of appetite booster. They described it as particularly cruel to trick Lilli's body into thinking it was hungry when all the other systems were telling her not to eat as a result of the transplant. Lilli did not eat anything for over a month, except for a few small pieces of ice. She claimed not to have an appetite and that everything we tried to feed her tasted awful, side effects of the transplant. The transplant team approached nutrition differently, by providing patients with bags of nutrition, TPN, during their stay in 5200 and then weaning patients off TPN if possible prior to discharge, transitioning to feeding tubes supplied with PediaSure from cans.

Lilli didn't take to the NG tube very easily, as she threw it up out of her mouth several times before she was finally able to keep it down. The nurses assured us that this was typical for patients not used to having feeding tubes. Once Lilli was finally able to keep down a tube, she tolerated it just enough since it was a ticket out of the hospital. We did our best to feed her through the tube as instructed and to continue the TPN also every night while Lilli slept.

Once Lilli was totally off the TPN, which meant that the team had confidence that she could get her own nutrition through a combination of the NG tube with PediaSure and the little bites that she started to eat, beginning with eggs and pasta, she began to take in more calories from the feeding tube. The feeding tube, however, started to bother Lilli, and she began to gag on the tube going down her throat. This hit a turning point one night when Lilli couldn't sleep because of her gagging and throwing up. We had to do something about it.

We called the clinic, and they sent us to the Jimmy Valvano Day Clinic the following day, on a weekend. Lilli was observed there by one of the clinic nurses we didn't know very well, and after some deliberation she came to the exam room and said, "I think we're just going to take out the NG tube and see what happens." She told Lilli that her nose and throat might burn for a day or two but that she would probably get some relief from not having the tube stuck down her nose. Instead of replacing the tube, the team decided to see if Lilli could get enough calories without the feeding tube. They suggested that Lilli could try to drink the shakes that we had left. Lilli was not a fan of those shakes, but her brother Collin couldn't get enough of them.

Lilli had lost a few pounds by that ninth week post-transplant. The feeding tube had taken its toll on her body, and she couldn't get enough calories from all the gagging and throwing up. Because of her weight loss, Lilli was put back on a daily clinic schedule. My summer studio had wrapped up, and I was able to help LouAnne get Lilli to the clinic on this daily routine. As a precaution, we had to draw more vials of blood each morning for additional tests.

Lilli had a different setback that week with her adrenal glands, which had been beaten and battered by her prolonged dependence on the steroids that kept her new cells in check. LouAnne took Lilli for her clinic appointment one day when I stayed at the RMH, and Erika, the nurse practitioner, took one look at her and said, "You need a stress dose of hydrocortisone. Your adrenal glands are suffering from the prednisone." Lilli had gone to the clinic that day exhausted and suffering, but the dose of hydrocortisone did the trick to revive her adrenal glands. The team adjusted a few of Lilli's prescriptions to address this new side effect to a side effect. The whole recovery period seemed like a balancing act of medications and procedures, and Lilli had a number of tweaks to this balance that week.

The medications that kept Lilli alive also came with a myriad of side effects. When we first met with Dr. Martin, even before Lilli finished treatments at Brenner, he mentioned the cyclosporine hair. He said, "Oh, you'll know when the cyclosporine kicks in." Later, after Lilli was admitted to 5200, I saw exactly what they were talking about. The post-transplant patients had puffy faces covered in dark, fuzzy peach-like hair. Girls and boys had moustaches, uni-brows, chin hair, sideburns, basically hair everywhere that a normal child would not have hair. Lilli's hair started growing back like this before she was discharged from 5200. She started growing hair in all those places, as a result of the anti-rejection drugs like cyclosporine and tacrolimus that she later took.

Lilli doesn't look like her old self, but at least she's alive. She looks like all those other transplant kids. I do hope this hair wears off soon, though, because teenagers can be cruel. I guess we'll find out who her true friends are.

Day +70

....

After a week when Lilli had a few bumps in the road to recovery, I was pleased to have a few positive developments. Lilli's blood counts had remained on an uphill trajectory towards normal, and her White Blood Count (WBC) was in the normal range for at least a week. Assuming that the donors' cells were still winning the battle for bone marrow dominance, these steady numbers were a relief. The hemoglobin and platelet numbers, while not yet in the normal range, were steadily increasing towards normal.

Our home healthcare made a turn for the better after all the challenges of the previous week. The number of pumps that we had to juggle every night decreased from four to one. The TPN, or Total Parenteral Nutrition, was discontinued due to some of Lilli's lab numbers. The feeding tube was removed after all the gagging, and I can't say that I regretted seeing it go. Lilli was free from the feeding tube, feeding pump, IV pole, and PediaSure, and she understood the pressure to get more calories and to try to drink some of the PediaSure shakes the old-fashioned way.

It was like Lilli flipped a mental switch when she had to start eating. She regained her appetite. She started eating three meals a day, and she even found an appetite for fast food. She dressed up one day to go out for a double cheeseburger from a drive-thru. While trying to get in better shape, I tried to swear off fast food, but for Lilli's sake I was happy for her to get high calorie meals, fat and sugar and all. She started gaining weight, replacing about two of the four pounds that she lost from the feeding tube struggles.

More good news came in the form of updates on the BK virus and quick clinic visits. The blood cultures from the night at the BOP had not grown anything, and the BK virus turned out to be a mild case that Lilli's body was fighting with the help of additional fluids. The clinic team was quite happy with the progress Lilli was making, the weight she was gaining, and the food that she was eating. They didn't keep Lilli long at the clinic; we got in and out in record time.

By the time week ten rolled around, the BK virus was in our rear-view mirror. Lilli was again the perfect post-transplant patient, and she was able to spread out her clinic appointments once again. Her blood counts continued to stabilize. Lilli was like her old self, dressing up in chic outfits and sunglasses to go to the clinic. I admired how she was able to stay so positive and upbeat in spite of all the things she endured through the treatment and recovery processes, and I fed off her strength and optimism.

On Sundays at the Ronald McDonald House, we could count on a visit from Stoel, one of my colleagues from UNCG who lived in Chapel Hill. Stoel and I had been teaching together for about six years by the time Lilli had her transplant, and most of my fondest memories of UNCG involved Stoel. We had taken students on a field trip to Chicago to compete in a skyscraper design competition, where our students did quite well. We had collaborated on the design of a solar powered house for the 2013 Solar Decathlon in support of Team Tidewater from Hampton and Old Dominion universities. And we had driven a van of students to Princeton, New Jersey, to visit my old boss and mentor Michael Graves who was by that time confined to a wheelchair after being paralyzed from a sinus infection that went to his brain.

Stoel was generous with his time as a colleague, and he was generous with his time and money as he delivered a wagon full of groceries to the RMH on Sunday afternoons. Occasionally Lilli would be able to get up and walk to the lobby to greet Stoel, but generally he would call when he got close to Durham and then knock on our apartment door with a wagon full of drinks and snacks in tow. The staff at the Ronald McDonald House grew to expect his visits and referred to him as the "wagon guy."

Though we didn't have many visitors at the RMH, Stoel wasn't the only friend to stop by. One Saturday morning, Lilli's Girl Scout troop from Greensboro came to Durham to make breakfast for the house. While Lilli still had to wear a mask around her friends and not hug them, she was able to come down from our suite to the kitchen to hang out with her friends. That morning I had gone for a run around the campus, and I returned to a breakfast of sausage and pancakes and grapes that Lilli's friends and Scout leader, Miss Kay, had prepared.

Lilli continued having good clinic appointments after that weekend. The team mentioned that Lilli would be on a typical plan for weekend passes for three or four weeks, and it would be less than a week before Lilli could go home for a pass. The team also informed us about a new battery of tests, similar to the tests that Lilli had before her transplant, to confirm the success of her transplant and to check her vital organs for any negative impacts from the transplant. It was still four weeks away, but for the first time we had a possible date for Lilli to be released to go home to Greensboro for good: August 29, 2016.

Asbestos at +77

When the social worker first interviewed LouAnne, Lilli, and me
before Lilli could qualify for her transplant, she asked us questions
about our family situation, our stability, our home life, and the
state of our house. Did we have a stable family? Did we argue a lot?
Did Lilli have her own room, or did she share a room? Did Lilli
have her own bed? Was the home safe? Did the house have mold
and mildew? Was it clean? I realized then that, although medically
Lilli was in need of a bone marrow transplant, the team couldn't
sign off on a transplant if Lilli were not being cared for socially,
emotionally, and psychologically. While the medical part was out
of our hands and in the hands of some of the most brilliant
oncologists on the planet, the other pieces were partially in our
control. I wanted to ask the social worker how in the world she
expected a patient with a life-threatening illness like Lilli's to have
a totally perfect home life, but I held my tongue, guessing that we'd
have to answer the questions without sass in order for the interview
to go smoothly.

As it got closer to the time for Lilli to go home for good, I started to worry about the basement in our house. Basements are notorious for growing mold and mildew and for harboring fungi that could be fatal to someone recovering from a bone marrow transplant. I decided that the smart thing to do would be to pull up the carpeting from the finished portion of our basement, roughly half of the basement, and replace it with something harder and more durable. At first, I thought that bamboo would be the perfect option; however, I learned that local installers would not certify a floor done in bamboo in a basement or other area below ground. Although our finished basement is a walk-out basement that has not flooded in the nine years we've lived there, I could see their point. Plan B was to go with a less sustainable vinyl plank with a wood finish in the den and office and to go with a porcelain tile in the laundry room and bathroom.

One evening when the rest of the family was in Durham at the RMH, I decided to go to Greensboro and start pulling up the carpet. I thought that I could at least do that part of the project myself. As I pulled up a few corners of the carpet, however, I came across something that looked suspiciously like asbestos tile from the 1960s. As an architect, I've had some experience working on older building renovations and have learned some of the telltale signs of vinyl tile containing asbestos, a naturally-occurring fire-resistant but cancer-causing mineral that was used extensively in building products like floor and ceiling tiles and siding well into the 1960s when our house was built. The first sign was the size of the tile. The older tiles are usually 9" squares, not the 12" squares currently used. The second sign was the black color of the mastic, another giveaway. While undisturbed asbestos can be sealed and considered safe, the chipping and cracking tile edges that I had exposed by pulling up the carpet gave me pause.

How did we get so lucky as to be living on top of a carcinogen? We can't afford to get rid of this tile properly. And we can't afford NOT to get rid of this!

Previous owners clearly covered over this asbestos tile, knowingly or unknowingly, with carpet and tack strips that caused the tile to fracture and potentially put our whole family at risk of contracting cancer from the asbestos. I couldn't risk it. I wasn't about to bring Lilli back into a house that could cause her to have a new cancer after spending over two years trying to save her life from cancer.

We had to act quickly to do something about the tile. I first called an environmental testing agency to have them send someone out to test samples from the tile and glue mastic. Those results came back a day or two later, and the amount of asbestos in the tile and mastic was higher than the testing guy had predicted. There was 5% asbestos in the 9x9 tile, and there was 8% asbestos in the black mastic. What luck! Finding asbestos in our house would've been a big deal anytime, but having this happen just weeks before a cancer survivor was scheduled to move back in was an emergency.

I then contacted a local demolition company that provides asbestos abatement services and a second company that specializes in asbestos abatement. Representatives from each of the companies came out to take a look at our basement and provided me with estimates. I explained to each of the men our situation, that Lilli was a cancer survivor who had just been cleared to return home following her transplant. One of the men sensed our urgency and had the capacity to start on the project almost immediately, and we agreed to proceed with the work as soon as we could clear out the basement. Our basement had not been empty since the night we moved into our brick ranch in 2010.

We had never cleared out our basement as quickly as we did that following weekend. I orchestrated the delivery of a pod container to our driveway and a crew of neighbors and church members to help move our things from the basement out to the pod on a Saturday morning. While I still wound up having to work into the wee hours of the night to clear out everything from the basement— except the toilet and lavatory—we managed to meet the abatement team's schedule to begin the project.

Yet again I got to experience crews of people decked out in hazmat suits. The last time I had seen those kinds of suits was in the hospital when Lilli had fevers or some undetected virus that she was fighting. And here was a crew of people cleaning out the cancer-causing material from our basement. They worked quickly and efficiently, taping and sealing off our basement from other areas of the house, then installing box fans in multiple windows to create negative air pressure to suck out whatever air particles they happened to stir up in the process. They proceeded by spraying chemicals on the asbestos-containing materials and scraping off the tile and mastic, exposing a bare concrete slab to match our unfinished basement floor. They removed bags full of tile and scrapings from their work in thick plastic hazmat bags that they taped up, hauled to the front of our house, and placed in their work truck. The crew had also installed an airlock at the basement door connected to a shower that they used to sanitize themselves before heading home. The crew left our home the way they found it, minus the flooring and mastic, exposing a bare concrete floor that remained damp for a few days. I went out and bought some box fans to run at high speed around the clock.

The lengths to which we had to go to provide a safer home for Lilli and the rest of our family were probably greater than we would have done without having gone through our ordeal with leukemia; however, the benefits of living without asbestos were invaluable. We could sleep at night knowing that we did our best, and with licensed experts, to remove the known cancer-causing flooring from our house. We then had the flooring replaced after allowing the space to air out for several days following an air test that showed a level of clean air that met federal and state guidelines. While all of this was going on, I stayed in the house while the rest of the family lived in the Ronald McDonald House an hour away.

The costs of Lilli's treatments meant that we had nothing in savings to pay for a new floor. We got some help from family members to pay for the asbestos removal, but we needed to apply for store credit at Lowe's Home Improvement to be able to pay for a new floor in our basement. I stayed in Greensboro for a few days to sort out the new flooring and to coordinate with the installers while LouAnne and the kids stayed at the RMH in Durham along with my sister Tammy. One evening LouAnne and I had a romantic date to Lowe's Home Improvement, making the most of the limited hours we had alone. We made flooring selections based on this quick trip to Lowe's together followed by my doing the best I could to roll with some of the changes due to availability and schedule. We had to take what we could get quickly and what was appropriate to use in a basement. With all that in mind I made the final selections, got approved for store credit (a blessing, considering how poor our finances were), and worked with the installers to coordinate the installation.

After getting past our emergency situation, we wound up with a durable and cleanable floor, one that would not trap dust and germs, that would last for years to come. The asbestos was gone, and the new floor was in. We called on our group of friends to help move all the furniture back inside from the driveway pod. This process also gave us a chance to cull some of the furniture that we had dreamed of getting rid of for years and to declutter our lives. This decluttering paled in comparison, however, to the number of plastic bins full of paperwork and arts and crafts that we had accumulated from two different hospitals.

Day +84

Nearing Day +100, Lilli was able to go home for a weekend pass around Day +84. We milked it for all it was worth, returning back to the RMH at 11:59PM Sunday night, just in time to get some sleep before heading back to the clinic on Monday morning for a check-up. The weekend pass meant that we didn't have to draw labs for a few days and could breathe a little bit during the mornings. As we talked to other patients' families, we heard stories about patients who had to stay longer than the 100 days post-transplant, and I hoped that we would be able to leave on or before the 100-day mark.

It was great to be in the same house as a family of five again. We all slept in our old beds again. I had replaced all our mattresses the previous summer when Lilli was discharged from Brenner, and in one year we had already worn grooves into our beds. Lilli and Amelia were back sleeping in the room at the opposite end of the

311

hall from ours, and Collin was back where he belonged, in the middle hallway bedroom. LouAnne and I were able to share a bed again in the privacy of our own room. We all ate meals around our old dining room table. The kids played games together. They enjoyed the newly straightened and cleaned basement with its new floor. And they picked on each other and argued with the same sibling rivalry they had from years before Lilli's cancer diagnosis.

The weekend was precious yet short-lived. We had to return to the Ronald McDonald House by Monday morning so that Lilli could report to the clinic to make sure that we had not broken her while on our weekend pass. I started teaching the day after we returned from our first weekend pass. Lilli was still at least 15 days from coming home for good, and I had just begun another fall semester. Time kept ticking, and I kept teaching. I had to plan my classes from the hospital clinic and the Ronald McDonald House, but I maintained a full-time teaching load. I commuted from Durham to Greensboro, from the Ronald McDonald House to my studio and lecture course at UNCG, every Tuesday and Thursday. In retrospect, I'm not sure how I did it, but I relied on muscle memory and many years of teaching experience.

I didn't take time off during Lilli's treatments. I was still a tenure-track faculty member in need of tenure to have job security. Lilli's cancer diagnosis had given me a more balanced view of my profession in relation to my family, but securing tenure at a public university would be a key to job security, continuity of health insurance, and some peace of mind about my family's future.

I had turned in my tenure dossier in several different PDFs from the hospital when Lilli was still on the 5200 unit as well as from the sofa of the Ronald McDonald House. I posted the files online, and they were being reviewed by my colleagues around the time that the Fall 2016 Semester began. I hoped and prayed that I would be awarded tenure and promoted to associate professor, but there was no guarantee. Time would tell. In the meantime, I continued to be a home health provider to my daughter, a father to three children, a husband who often slept in a different bed from my wife, and a full-time professor and university research center director.

Day +91

During Lilli's second weekend back in Greensboro on a weekend pass she had a slight bump in the road to recovery in the form of stomach-bug-like symptoms. She threw up and had a sore stomach for several days. LouAnne and I worried that these symptoms marked the return of a more serious Graft-vs-Host flare-up, but her labs didn't indicate any GVH. Two of the three main indicators in Lilli's blood were in the normal range, and overall her bone marrow was functioning.

We tempted fate by packing up a few of our things from the Ronald McDonald House and driving them home to Greensboro. We had books, toys, food, pots, pans, clothes, boxes, bins, and cleaning products. We had a ton of cleaning products at the RMH. We had to worry about cleanliness wherever we went, and we had accumulated all kind of wipes, sprays, liquids, bottles, and canisters. We had gotten in the habit of wiping clean the toilet and shower and sink after every time one of us used them, as Lilli needed to have the cleanest surfaces touching her skin. We had hospital-grade wipes that, along with the pumps and meds, came home with us. We were not the most rigorous in cleaning our home before Lilli's transplant, but afterwards, we had become obsessive about germs.

My sister, Tammy, helped us sanitize our home in preparation for Lilli's return. Tammy decided to accept an early retirement from her school system in South Georgia, which meant that she could spend more time helping us that summer after Lilli's transplant. She scrubbed and scrubbed on our old 1960 brick ranch's bathrooms and kitchen. Part of our asbestos abatement and removal included replacing the plumbing fixtures in our downstairs half bathroom. That bathroom wasn't nearly as dirty as the older ones, but Tammy had to work extra hard to sanitize our older bathrooms.

At the clinic, Lilli's team remained impressed by her progress. They continued to talk about Day +100, perhaps earlier, as the day to release Lilli back to her primary oncology team at Brenner Children's Hospital. Lilli had additional labs drawn in preparation for her Day +100 work-up. The team would look at those lab results the following week to determine how successful the transplant was. Lilli would also prepare for the additional tests that the team would review as we approached Day +100. The regular labs that I was drawing in the mornings continued to improve, and now two of the three primary markers were in the "normal" range. What a relief! It had been two months without any blood or platelet transfusions nor white blood cell booster drugs, all signs that Lilli's bone marrow was functioning.

In preparation for Lilli's homecoming, the team discontinued her IV fluids at home. We were down from four pumps at home to *zero* pumps. There were still plenty of prescription medications for Lilli to take and for us to manage, but it was like Christmas morning when we didn't have to connect any more pumps at home. The portable IV pole that Lilli had dragged around every day and night at the RMH could finally go back in its box and be stored in the closet. The daily deliveries of refrigerated fluids from the pharmacy to the Ronald McDonald House stopped, and we got several hours of our lives back each day.

In exchange for the freedom from IV nutrition and fluids, Lilli had to track her calorie and fluid intakes. With her love of spreadsheets, schedules, and planners, Lilli welcomed the opportunity to track her diet. Armed with her smart phone and laptop, Lilli researched the menus of her favorite restaurants and their published calorie counts. While I was watching my diet, and trying to reduce my calorie intake, Lilli was looking for foods and meals that could provide large numbers of calories for weight gain.

Day +98

Two days shy of the 100-day benchmark, that mythical number, LouAnne, Lilli, and I met with the transplant team at Duke. Most of the results from the 100-day lab study drawn the previous week were back, and Lilli's primary transplant doctor used the phrase "almost too good to be true," to describe some of the counts. One of those counts was Lilli's ALC, or Absolute Lymphocyte Count. While we had focused so much time and energy on Lilli's ANC, or Absolute Neutrophil Count, I had been distracted from worrying about the number of lymphocytes floating around in Lilli's body. Given the root of Lilli's leukemia in her myeloid cells and not her lymphocytes, I had not given a lot of thought to lymphocytes. The team reminded us that lymphocytes, while not as prominent a marker of bone marrow and immune system recovery as the neutrophil count, were still a marker to monitor. Lilli's lymphocytes had begun an upward trajectory and indicated a faster-than-normal recovery for Lilli's bone marrow.

The chimerism labs, showing how much of Lilli's old DNA remained (or didn't), were rock solid again. With no guarantee, ever, that Lilli's old cells wouldn't come back, I exhaled a sigh of relief that the 100-day labs still showed no trace of Lilli's old DNA in her blood. The team said that they would re-do the chimerism labs at Lilli's annual check-up each year and that there was no guarantee that the cells from Donor #2's cord blood would continue to win out. We were all encouraged by the results.

The previous week, Lilli had to go through a whole battery of tests like the ones she had done in order to qualify for the bone marrow transplant. This time the tests were like her final exams. The team went over the results of those tests with us and let us know, generally-speaking, the effect that the transplant had on Lilli's vital organs. I paid attention to Lilli's doctor as he went through page after page of numbers, data, percentages, charts, and graphs, but it all became a blur. What stood out to me was the number of times we read the word "normal" in the written description of Lilli's individual parts.

Normal heart.

Normal liver.

Normal kidneys.

Normal chest.

Normal range for lungs.

Dr. Martin pointed out that the minor damage to Lilli's lungs meant that she'd never be a world-class sprinter, distance runner, or endurance athlete, and Lilli was okay with that result. She didn't have any aspirations for gold medals in any sport. While I wished that the transplant would be a true cure-all and that Lilli's body would be back to perfect, I accepted the impact that the procedures and recovery had on my daughter in exchange for her being able to live a longer life. She would've been dead without the life-saving medical advances in using umbilical cord blood stem cells.

There we were at Day +98. It was two days before that mythical 100th day post-transplant. We had gone on an incredible journey to move to a summer home in Durham at the Ronald McDonald House while maintaining our home and jobs in Greensboro the entire time. I didn't know in April when we packed up Lilli's stuff and drove to Durham whether or not she would return with us in 100 days or if our time would be cut short. We were about to hear the best news we had heard all year. Dr. Martin said, "Lilli, we're going to release you back home and to the oncology team at Brenner. You're more than welcome to come back here since you are our patient, but we're happy to turn you over to Dr. Buckley."

I wanted to cry, but there were no tears that day, only joy and smiles. Lilli was beaming with pride. LouAnne and I looked at each other and smiled. I couldn't believe our good fortune with Lilli's transplant and recovery, and we were about to go home for good to reconnect as a family of five.

Before we could leave the clinic, however, the team had a few things for Lilli. Since it was a week before her 14th birthday, the team brought Lilli a few gifts to the exam room. More of the staff came in to the room to join in singing a round of *Happy Birthday* to Lilli. How great it was to see grown men and women (with watery eyes) who had taken care of our girl for four months singing a song and sending us off to be a normal family once again!

That afternoon we took home a lot of paperwork with plenty of instructions. Lilli was still restricted from going out in public. She could be with us at home, in the hospital, or outdoors, but she still couldn't go back to school, church, restaurants, stores, or other enclosed public spaces. She would have to report to her primary oncology team at Brenner each week for blood draws and a physical check-up. And we would have to take her to the surgical unit at the hospital to have Lilli's central line removed after a few weeks. Lilli would be able to re-register for school in our home district, but she wouldn't be able to go back to school for many months. All those restrictions, however, could not steal the joy that I felt on Day +98 when the team at Duke finally gave us permission to go home.

Lilli Owl Socks

....

Shortly after Lilli was released to go home to Greensboro,
LouAnne took her for one of her first check-ups back at Brenner
in Winston-Salem. While they were there, the social worker
approached LouAnne about a new initiative started by an adult
bone marrow transplant patient who was in college for business
and entrepreneurship at Wake Forest University. The social
worker described an opportunity for Lilli to design a sock, as the
college student named Jake was starting a small business to help
cancer patients design their own socks to raise money. Jake's story
was compelling, and I trusted him to honor and respect Lilli and
our family throughout the process.

The sock design process sounded like a great idea to LouAnne and
Lilli, and I agreed that it would be a great experience for any
teenager. While we had gone through several t-shirt fundraisers
with #LilliSTRONG and a year later #LilliSTRONGER on the
shirts, Lilli now had an opportunity to leave her mark in sock

drawers around the world. In the past, the t-shirts and wristbands had been designed by others, incorporating Lilli's favorite colors and owls. Lilli weighed in with a thumbs-up when she liked the t-shirt designs. This time, Lilli would be able to do the design work herself.

Jake called and described his vision for his business which started as a result of his winning a campus student contest, similar to the one we have at UNCG for business students, the Minute-to-Win-It shark-tank presentation for which there's some modest prize money. Jake was turning his student project into a real business endeavor called Resilience Gives. He had collaborated with student filmmakers and designers to start this sock design company, and he was looking for pediatric patients to volunteer to work with him. Lilli was excited by the prospect of designing a sock.

Jake and his graphic designer colleague came out to our house to visit with Lilli, LouAnne, and me on a weekday when Amelia and Collin were in school. Jake asked Lilli about her favorite colors for the socks and talked through the concept of putting owls on the socks. Would it be one great big owl to cover the entire sock? Would it be a lot of tiny owls in a graphic pattern? Lilli suggested that they use one or two medium-sized owls in a field of color, and the graphic designer got to work. I asked Lilli if she wanted to sketch anything herself, but her approach to design was to search online for typical owl designs and to choose a handful of those designs to forward to Jake's graphic designer who worked back-and-forth via e-mail and text with Lilli to arrive at the final design of the socks, the *Lilli Owl*.

Once the sock design was set, Jake and his team worked on sourcing the socks and the distribution system. Since Lilli's design was only the second sock that Resilience had done, Jake was doing much of the packaging and shipping himself. I was impressed by the amount of care and attention he gave to packaging and branding.

Prior to releasing the socks for sale, Jake and a team of videographers came to our house to interview Lilli and our family for a video segment to promote sales. With the owl theme of Lilli's socks, the team turned our living room into an owl's nest by hanging a lot of Lilli's stuffed owls on our curtains as a backdrop to the video. We talked about the cost of cancer and transplant treatments and about how the sock sales would help defray the high costs of cancer. The video joined other videos in Jake's collection of marketing materials that helped to tell his story about how his love of crazy socks helped him through his own bone marrow transplant.

We announced the socks to our friends and family, and our supporters couldn't wait to get their hands on Lilli's socks. Many of those in our community wanted to help us with our finances, and a pair of socks was a tangible thing that folks could wear while supporting us financially. The design was launched just before Christmas 2016 during Lilli's eighth grade year, and many of our friends and family got socks for Christmas that year. Each pair of socks wrapped in tissue paper came packaged in a custom box with a photo of Lilli, a description of the *Lilli Owl*, and a blank card for buyers to write an encouraging note to Lilli.

Jake coordinated a TV shoot at our home with a local news crew around the time the socks launched. Lilli had become used to making appearances on local television, having appeared a few times during her cancer treatments. I had a connection with one of the local newscasters because of some work my students had previously done with tiny houses for addressing homelessness in Greensboro. I reached out to that contact when I saw the Katy Perry video that Lilli's school had done, and they ran a piece on their afternoon news about that video. Later, they returned to our home to interview us about how the school had helped Lilli stay on top of her school work through the use of technology. They came back to do a piece on Lilli's sock designs as part of a larger segment about Jake and Resilience Gives. The local paper also ran an article about Lilli's sock design and how it connected to Jake's business.

Lilli still considers the *Lilli Owl* socks as a highlight of her journey through leukemia. Socks are still available through Resilience Gives, but the designs have evolved of the years. While our family no longer receives a portion of the proceeds from sock sales, Jake has expanded his business to support even more families and patients who are going through cancer treatments, in collaboration with a nonprofit based in Boston. This organization, Family Reach, has supported our family in recent years with financial assistance and financial planning, as the financial effects of cancer treatments on our family will last for many years.

Cannonball Run

After successfully running a half marathon distance on my own one day when Lilli was at Duke, I was confident that I'd be able to run that distance in a race. I looked online, again, and I discovered that the Cannonball Half Marathon was going to be run along my normal route in Greensboro. I signed up for the half marathon and continued training as normal. While there were plenty of half marathon training plans online, I didn't have the time or discipline to stick to a training plan like those. My friend Andy crafted a plan for me, but I couldn't keep up with that one, either.

When race day came around I was nervous, but I didn't have far to drive, merely a mile from door to starting line. I still didn't know how to warm up, but there was a guided warm up session in the parking lot of Country Park where the race started. The race organizers had planned for everything, as far as I could tell, including a mobile stage complete with sound system for the trainers who ran the warm-up session.

I had no idea what pace I would run, as it was only the third time I had run the 13.1-mile distance, but I looked for the 2:00 pacers and the 1:45 pacers. I figured that I was somewhere between those two projected finish times. A day earlier, when I picked up my race packet at the nearby Omega Sports, I bumped into my running friend, Jonathan, from church. He introduced me to Thad McLaurin, a local running coach known as the *Runner Dude*, who advised me to "Start out in the slower pacing group, and aim to catch up with the faster pacing group along the way if you're able. You can't win the race in the first few miles, but you can lose it by going out too fast."

I pondered that advice plus the other advice that Jonathan gave me via text: "Use Gold Bond powder and two large round band-aids."

I understand the talcum powder, but where am I supposed to put the band-aids? Are they for back-up down there, in case the powder doesn't work? That would really hurt when I go to pull them off. That can't be right. I think I'll just stick with what got me here...nothing down my shorts, and pray for the best.

I started off a little in front of the 2:00 pacers but with the 1:45 pacers still in sight. It wasn't long before I lost sight of the 1:45 pacers and their sign on a stick. After looping around the lakes at Country Park and heading back up and around Lawndale Road to come back around to near where we started, I had run the first few miles without knowing my pace. Although I had started the running app on my phone, I didn't want to pull the phone from my armband. It was just too hard to take it out and then put it back without a lot of effort while on the run. Instead, I found a runner who was keeping my same pace and asked what our pace was. He looked at his watch, let me know that we were running somewhere around an 8:05/mile pace, and said that if I could stick with him then he'd bring me in at the finish line around 1:48. This sounded like a good plan to me, but I didn't have enough experience to know if I could sustain that pace for all 13.1 miles.

This other runner, a guy named Mark from Virginia, and I talked and ran together for the next three or four miles. I gave him some important reconnaissance information about the route, as it was my everyday route, up the Atlantic and Yadkin Greenway, past the Guilford Courthouse battleground site, past Lake Brandt towards Bur Mil, and back. At around mile five or six Mark pulled out something from his running belt, squeezed it in his mouth, and then took a swig of water from one of his water bottles clipped to his belt.

I asked him, "What was that?"

"Gel," he responded, and proceeded to tell me all about nutrition for a half marathon versus nutrition for a full marathon. I had never heard of energy gels, and I definitely didn't train for my first half marathon with any gels. I also didn't carry my own water. Instead, I picked up a bottle of water from a water station a short distance from Mark's beautifully executed gel-water combo without missing a step. I struggled to drink the water while running, a skill that I had never even tried, as I had not been training with water.

I kept up with Mark, even as our pace slowed to around 8:25/mile going uphill towards Owl's Roost Rd, and then I held on for dear life as we ran downhill towards the pond near Bur Mil. When we reached the halfway point, I had to slow down and let Mark run ahead at his own pace. I grabbed a cup of water around that time and proved that I had never drunk from a cup of water while running…ever. A pro tip for anyone who's planning on drinking from a paper or plastic cup during a race is to pinch the middle of the top of the cup, making a little spout in one edge of the cup, and then sip from that spout. Instead, I kept running while trying to drink from the unmodified lip of the cup, nearly choking on a sip of water that went both in my mouth and (mostly) up my nose. I coughed and wheezed while simultaneously struggling to keep pace anywhere nearly as fast as Mark and I started.

It was at the uphill pond climb portion of the greenway when I lost my energy and snorted a water cup. I struggled to keep running up the hill, but I did keep running for a while. I managed to make it up one of the hardest hills around mile 9 or 10 and had a downhill section that gave me a chance to dwell on the upcoming hill beside the Food Lion on Lawndale. While I had never run that hill, neither up nor down, I could visualize it in my mind.

Oh, wait! That Food Lion hill's going to be a killer. If I'm running down this steep hill right now, then I'm about to pay for it when I turn the corner. I'm not gonna be able to keep running.

My fears were realized when I turned the corner at Lawndale and saw what may as well have been Mt. Everest. I couldn't keep running up that hill, and the sad part was that once I walked to the top of that hill there were several more uphill sections. I should've studied the race's section diagram more carefully and should've saved some of my energy for the final 3-4 miles. I needed every bit of grit I could muster to make it from the Food Lion to the finish line.

Over the final stretch, I was the target for other runners to pick off as they passed me on their way to faster finishes. I felt both pride for running as long as I had and shame for crashing, or bonking, at the end of the race and having to run-walk the final three-mile rolling hills stretch around Country Park. The race finished on a steep uphill.

Thanks a lot, race organizers! Who puts a hill at the end of a half marathon!?

I had just enough energy left at the end to run the final tenth of a mile, and I finished with a time of 1:54:38, which was in the range I hoped to hit. I came in 12th place for men in my age group, but I was disappointed that I couldn't run the entire race.

To redeem myself, I looked for another half marathon in my area. Within a few days after the Cannonball Half, I found the Mayberry Half Marathon—named after the Andy Griffith hometown—held in Mount Airy, NC, the following month. I trained a bit for that race, but there wasn't much time for a complete training program. I had run the first half marathon without using any plan, which gave me the confidence that I could run the Mayberry Half without following a plan. A friend at church who heard that I was going to run that race gasped, "I ran that one, and it's Hilly! Good luck with that!"

OK? I guess the race is going to have a lot of hills. It is in Mount Airy, which is literally a town on a mountain known for Andy Griffith and its granite quarries. Oh well, I don't know whether to believe the advertising for the race, saying that it's flat and fast, or my friend who said it was hilly. I'll just have to be ready for whatever comes my way.

I drove up to Mount Airy the night before the race, and Amelia volunteered to ride with me. It was in November, and it was dark before we got to town to pick up the race bib and t-shirt packet. In the dark, I couldn't get my bearings and figure out exactly where the race would start, but I trusted that I was close enough to the start line and could find my way there the following day.

In the morning, I drove myself up to the Mount Airy address in the race packet, a parking lot near a park and greenway. I had not run many races at all, but this was my first race with a bus shuttle that took runners to the starting line. I hopped on the bus with other runners, and we rode uphill (a good sign, because it meant we'd be running downhill at some point) to Main Street and the starting line. I got my nervous jitters out by jogging around and trying to do some dynamic stretches on my own.

I had learned a few things from the Virginian runner Mark during the Cannonball Half Marathon, and those lessons revolved around hydration, nutrition, and pacing. After that embarrassing run-in with a cup of water during my first half marathon, I decided to buy a handheld water bottle for runners, one with a built-in hand strap and zipper pocket. With water bottle in hand, I was able to stay hydrated during the race. I had trained with energy gels for a few weeks before the Mayberry Half, and I packed a few in the zipper compartment of my water bottle holder. Lastly, after struggling to run with my phone, I bought a GPS watch for runners to track my pace and distance in real time. I was ready for Mayberry.

The race didn't have a huge turnout, but there were enough runners for emotional support and encouragement along the 13.1-mile route. Heading down Main Street behind a classic Andy Griffith era police car pacer at the start of the race, the pack ran quickly downhill and back towards the parking lot where we picked up the shuttle bus. Maybe the advertisement was accurate, and this race would be flat and fast. After another quick turn, down and around the parking lot, we headed out onto an asphalt greenway that ran along a shallow creek. It was a chilly but clear fall day, and the sun shone through the red, orange, and yellow leaves that burned bright along the route.

I locked into step with a woman running just in front of me. I kept track of her by focusing on a distinctive hummingbird tattoo on her calf. For as long as I could keep up with her, I used the woman with the hummingbird tattoo as my pacer. While there were volunteer pacers for the 2:00 (approximately 9 minutes per mile) and 1:45 (approximately 8 minutes per mile) times, I was somewhere in-between and followed my unofficial pacer. My new GPS watch helped me know my pace, but I hadn't yet figured out that I could switch the display from the current real-time pace to a lap, or single mile, pace. My display was stuck on real-time pace, which meant that I didn't know my one mile splits until the end of each mile.

After running an 8:08/mile pace the first mile, I settled in behind the hummingbird-tattoo pacer who unknowingly paced me through a lot of evenly-paced miles of 8:05-8:10/mile. I stayed on her heels for half of the race, and then I passed her near the 7-mile turnaround, shortly after taking an energy gel to boost my carbs and sugar levels. With rolling hills of greenway that I had already run, in the opposite direction, I gained confidence that I could run a PR (Personal Record) if I could just hold it together.

For the mile after the turnaround, I picked up my pace a little, something I find myself doing in races when I am suddenly face-to-face with runners who are running just a few meters behind me. Once I settled back down to a more reasonable pace, I continued to run a strong race and enjoyed the beautiful scenery. I passed a few runners, and a few runners passed me, but I was still running. I had managed to run a better race than the Cannonball the previous month, but there were still a few more miles of the race when I started to feel exhausted. It would be a struggle to finish the final 2-3 miles anywhere near the pace I had established earlier. Around mile 11, the woman with the hummingbird tattoo passed me. "Good job," I told her. She was obviously better at pacing the entire race, where I still had to learn how to pace myself start-to-finish. I pulled out another energy gel in a panic, relying on anything and everything that could help me make it to the finish line.

The final two miles were a struggle. My pace decreased, and I fought an internal battle between the "stop-and-walk" doubts and the "you-can-do-this" affirmations. It was all I could do to keep running, as I passed a few runners who had stopped to walk. This was me in my previous half marathon where I had to stop and walk-run the final few miles. I dug deep to find the endurance to keep running, and I maintained a respectable pace over the final

5k. In the final mile, I knew I was getting close to the finish line. Runners who had already finished were walking back along the greenway to cheer other runners. I could hear the music and the crowd of finishers and supporters. I turned to run around the park and parking lot, and I saw the digital clock at the finish line.

Does that really say 1:48?? Is it possible for me to finish in under 1:50? Here I go!

I kicked it into high gear and sprinted to the finish. My official time was 1:49:16, just under an hour and fifty minutes. My second half marathon was a nearly perfect race for me, except for losing some steam near the end, and I could claim a PR after that one. Looking back at my one-mile splits, I could see how well the hummingbird tattoo pacer had helped me through the first half of the run. My splits were: 8:07, 8:18, 8:08, 8:08, 8:08, 8:16, 8:16, 8:07, 8:18, 8:35, 8:52, 8:51, 8:54 (6:59-sprint to finish). I never got her name, but I gave her a high five and told her, "Awesome race!" afterwards in the parking lot.

I was on a high after that race. Dreaming of running even faster half marathons, I couldn't wait to sign up for more races. I went home and researched more races in my area, but I waited until Christmas of 2016 to sign up for anything. Around that time there was a half marathon four-race special, offered by a local race organizer, called the *Half Crazy Series*. I signed up to run four half marathons in 2017 at a deep discount, and that race package was my big Christmas present that year. Now all I had to do was to continue to train and to be ready to run four half marathons, three in the spring and one in the fall of 2017.

Am I really crazy? Or am I just hooked on running half marathons? Either way, I'm in the best shape of my life and my lowest weight since grad school.

Hyperglycemia

I was in Washington, DC, for a training session for the National Architectural Accrediting Board (NAAB) in November 2016, NAAB is a volunteer third-party organization for which I volunteer to visit schools of architecture for the purpose of reviewing them for potential accreditation. Sitting at a round table in a windowless ballroom in the basement of a DC hotel, I got a text from LouAnne that she was at the oncology clinic with Lilli. Lilli had been struggling for a few days, losing energy and going pee a lot. We had suspected something for a few days when I had to go for this training. Although I didn't like to go out of town when Lilli was not well, she had been doing so well with her recovery and being weaned off the various post-transplant meds that I decided to accept the invitation for this mandatory training workshop.

Later that day I got word from LouAnne that Lilli had been admitted with high blood sugar levels, high enough that the doctors wanted to monitor her overnight and then put her on insulin until we could get her glucose levels under control. The cause of her high blood sugar was the continued use of steroids to keep the new donor's cells in check. Lilli had been taking prednisone regularly for over four months, and her body could not manage without having insulin injections. When LouAnne asked if this diabetes would be temporary or permanent, the doctors made us believe that once Lilli could be weaned off the steroids, then her glucose would drop down to a normal level.

Because I was out of town, LouAnne had to take Amelia and Collin to the hospital to spend the night, too. After their one-night sleepover in the hospital, though, Lilli was discharged. Everyone was home by the time I returned from DC. LouAnne and I had to learn a whole new set of home healthcare procedures at that point. We had to master new pieces of equipment, like a finger pricking tool, which Lilli ultimately mastered on her own, a diagnostic tool to digitally check and give a readout of the glucose level from little strips with drops of blood, and an old-fashioned syringe and needle with which to administer the insulin into Lilli's thigh muscles. At first, we struggled with the finger pricking procedure, as Lilli's fingers would often not bleed quite enough to register. She got frustrated by these new home health procedures that took some time to master.

I stressed about Lilli's high blood sugar levels, as a blood cancer was the start of our acute healthcare journey with Lilli. We had gone from worrying about Lilli's blood cells' containing cancerous cells to worrying about the sugar levels in her blood. I couldn't help but worry that there could be a connection between these two otherwise unrelated issues and that Lilli's cancer could return somehow because of what was going on with her diabetes, or hyperglycemia.

The daily home healthcare that LouAnne and I had to provide had gotten easier as Lilli was weaned off her huge list of transplant medications; however, the steroid-induced diabetes ratcheted up our parental responsibilities. We had to keep track of the insulin bottles stored in the refrigerator and had to monitor the numbers of test strips and syringes that we kept in the house. Lilli tracked her blood sugar counts, and we had to call in her counts to a nurse periodically. The nurse would ask us to adjust the dose of insulin based on Lilli's counts.

During the time when Lilli was on insulin, from November 2016 until January 2017, she remained puffy and hairy. The steroids that helped to keep the donor's cells in check came with side effects of high blood sugar and puffiness, particularly in Lilli's face. The hair that had come as a result of the cyclosporine, or anti-rejection medication, took months to wear off. Lilli still had bushy eyebrows, dark thick hair, and peach fuzz still on her face. She was virtually unrecognizable, yet she looked like almost all the other post-transplant patients whom we followed on social media. These patients could've passed for the same person at different points in time.

While Lilli managed a delicate recovery from her transplant and all its side effects, she was still an eighth grader who had to keep up with all her classes. She was in school, but she couldn't go inside the school building; instead, two of Lilli's friends carried her around the school. The staff set up a system for Skyping into class, and they made sure there was a dedicated laptop at the school for Lilli's virtual involvement. Lilli used a school-provided laptop at home to keep up with the online software used by the school, and Lilli used her own laptop, a gift from one of my childhood classmates, for the Skype video conferencing.

To keep up with school, Lilli had to wake up each school day the same as she would were she to go to school. She was responsible and independent in keeping up with this schedule. She would sit at her desk in her bedroom and follow along with the teachers' instruction. When I was her age, I might've looked for any excuse to get out of school, but Lilli fought hard to stay involved in her classes.

Once a week, the county's homebound teacher would come to our house to work with Lilli for an hour. To maintain her status in the school system, Lilli had to work with a homebound teacher, no matter what, and the teacher provided a connection to the outside world that Lilli desperately missed. Lilli connected much better with this second homebound teacher than the previous year's teacher.

Lilli still couldn't leave home to go to any public places for a long time. LouAnne and I had to provide around-the-clock home healthcare. Amelia and Collin provided companionship and amusement. The homebound situation at home was more difficult to manage than when Lilli was in the hospital. I was still teaching a full load at UNC Greensboro while running a research center on top of my teaching load. LouAnne was starting to get back to her normal schedule of teaching pre-school music. In spite of our career obligations, however, we were tethered to our home and to Lilli. When Lilli was in the hospital, we could depend on nurses and hospital staff to take care of her. But now, we were the doctors and nurses…and the professor, and the music teacher, and the husband and wife, and the parents to two other children.

I'm not sure any of our friends, family, or co-workers really got it. They saw that we were home, that Lilli was alive and recovering, and that we were managing to go back to work; however, I was more emotionally exhausted than ever. Running kept me in shape physically, and taking care of Lilli that year required all the physical fitness that running could provide.

A Year of Races

I stayed in shape by running and training for multiple races. I had one great physical after another with my primary care physician who said, "Just keep doing what you're doing." For my 2016 Christmas present I had gotten the privilege to endure four different half marathon races.

It's crazy how much money people will pay to suffer through 13.1 miles. And now I'm one of those crazy people!

It was also around Christmas 2016 when I learned through Facebook that one of the patients from 5200 who was there at the same time as Lilli had not been doing well. He was a few doors down and would sometimes walk up and down the hall at the same time as Lilli and I would walk. This teenager's parents wound up getting the news that I feared, that the doctors had done everything they could but that the cancer was just too strong and persistent to do anything else. I followed the family on Facebook to learn that shortly before New Year's 2017 this young man passed away from his cancer. Watching more young people die from cancer, I renewed my commitment to my own health in 2017.

The first half marathon I ran in 2017 was the Run Crystal Coast Half Marathon in Morehead City, NC, my third half marathon. After driving down to the coast of North Carolina the night before the race and having some car trouble along the way, I got to bed around midnight. It was hard for me to sleep with the wind whipping around the hotel tower and howling through the cracks in the room's sliding door leading to a balcony. Once I awoke and got dressed and ready to run, however, I felt great. I dressed in my cold weather running gear, showing off my new UNCG wicking t-shirt. I had vowed not to buy any UNCG-branded clothes until I was successful in securing tenure, and I had just been notified of my tenure and promotion to associate professor a few weeks before the race in Morehead City.

From the starting line beside the Morehead City Waterway, we ran through coastal neighborhoods a block or two from the water. I ran a pretty steady 10 miles of the race and was on pace to match my personal best until I...hit...that...bridge! Almost the entire course was as flat as a pancake, except for a bridge that we ran across near the beginning of the race. Going out over the bridge to Atlantic Beach around mile 2-3 was a piece of cake. Coming back over the bridge to Morehead City, against a headwind, around mile 10-11 was rough. I luckily made it over the bridge in one piece, still running, and finished with a time of 1:51:29, only two minutes slower than my best finish at the Mayberry Half.

At the Crystal Coast race, I continued my hydration and nutrition strategies that had worked at the Mayberry race, and I added one component to my training that my runner friend Jonathan talked about. He mentioned that his coach recommended coconut water for hydration before and after long runs and races, and he was hooked on it. I decided to give coconut water a chance, and I found some at my local grocery store. How expensive could coconut water be? Apparently, it's pretty expensive to hydrate with this stuff. I started with one carton, to see if I liked the taste, before looking for a case of it. I took home the carton of coconut water, poured a little in a glass, took a swig, and spit it out. Yuck! I imagined some native Pacific islander opening up a coconut, pouring out the coconut water into a dish, soaking his feet in this dish, and then pouring it into the carton from which I drank. I had rarely tasted anything as vile as coconut water, yet after enduring the bad taste for long enough to finish the expensive carton, I developed a tolerance and later a liking for this alternative sports drink.

The next half marathon I ran in 2017, half marathon #4, was the Hop Swap Half Marathon sponsored by the Foothills Brewery in Winston-Salem. I was looking forward to this springtime race because I would get to run in a different part of Winston-Salem, the city where Lilli and I had driven to the emergency room over two years before the race. I was still in great shape from regular training in Greensboro, a city with rolling and winding hills, but I was not entirely prepared for all the hills that Winston-Salem threw at me. Going from a table-top flat race at the coast to a very hilly race in the Piedmont-Triad was a shock. There was no way I could match the speed of my coastal race, but I finished in a respectable time of 1:53:48 and fourth place in my age group. The highlight of the race was my running into one of Lilli's oncologists from the hospital, Dr. McLean, the same doctor who called me one afternoon to say that Lilli's leukemia had most likely returned. He was not in the race, but he was cheering the runners from his front yard, where I first saw him, and later running in his neighborhood, where I passed him on my way back to the finish line.

After finding my groove with these half marathons, I decided to do something that I might advise others against. I had already signed up for the Carolina Brewsfest Half Marathon in High Point, NC, when the race organizers announced a special offer: Run the Brewsfest Half on Saturday AND the Run 13.1 in Greensboro on Sunday, and win a third medal for running two half marathons in the same weekend.

A THIRD MEDAL? Count me in! What's the worst thing that could happen? I might not finish the second race. I might not be able to run at all on Sunday. Even if I have to walk the second half marathon on Sunday, by God I'm going to do it.

I didn't announce to many people my plan to go crazy with two races in one weekend, but I found out after the second race that I wasn't the only person crazy enough to run two half marathons back-to-back. There was a pile of these special third medals lying on a table near the finish line.

The half marathon that Saturday in May was beautiful. I had never run in High Point, but I enjoyed the downtown start and finish with a long stretch of rolling greenway in the middle. It reminded me a lot of the greenway training that I did near my home. I maintained a steady pace throughout the race until a steep hill around miles 12-13. I figured out that race organizers must all go through the same training session when it comes to mapping out race routes. Just about every half marathon I had run came with a whopping hill or bridge near the end of the race. The Brewsfest in High Point was no exception. I slowed down with a mile left, but I found a higher gear near the finish when it looked like several runners might catch or pass me. I had a strong kick to the finish and had a time of 1:51:53, fifth place in my age group.

Immediately following the race, I drove to Kernersville where LouAnne and the kids were walking a 5k to raise money for the oncology unit at the children's hospital. I tried to get there in time to walk with them and our friends who teamed up with us, but they were finished walking by the time I arrived. I still got to catch up with some of our friends and some of the nurses and staff from the children's hospital. That afternoon, I rested as much as possible and prepared mentally to run another half marathon the following morning.

The Sunday morning half marathon started from a nearby shopping center and went through familiar neighborhoods. After the first mile or two, I realized that I could, in fact, still run in spite of running a half marathon the previous day. I didn't know if I could keep it up over the entire distance, but my goal shifted from "just finish" to "see if I can break two hours." The race organizers could've been professors of planning race routes, as they had found the hilliest streets and greenways available in town. I didn't struggle too much with the elevation on the way out, but in an out-and-back course I had to walk some of the hills on the way back to the shopping center finish line. Keeping an eye on my watch and my pace, I calculated that I had a fighting chance to stay under two

344

hours and to stay right around 9 minutes per mile. Walking some of the steep hills near the end of the race and nearly sprinting in between those hills, I finished the race in 1:56:46, exceeding my expectations and proving that I could run back-to-back races. I might have been crazy when I signed up for the challenge, but I walked away from that weekend with not two, but three medals for my hard work and dedication to fitness.

One Year Post-Transplant

As Lilli's one year transplant anniversary approached, LouAnne scheduled the requisite follow-up appointments at Duke. Although Lilli had been seen by the oncologists at Brenner on a bi-weekly basis during that year, she would need more extensive tests done at Duke. She would have to repeat the battery of tests that had established her baseline prior to transplant and that had been repeated around her Day +100.

In mid-May, LouAnne, Lilli, and I climbed in the car and drove to Durham for a day at the Duke bone marrow transplant clinic while Amelia and Collin were in school. We checked in at the 4th floor reception desk and then waited in chairs with a view towards the large atrium and the hustle of traffic and life outside the hospital. Lilli revealed her *Lilli Owl* socks as she crossed her legs, casually awaiting the labs and tests. I texted Lilli's hospital teacher, Josh, to let him know we would be there, and he said that he'd catch up with us later.

After the nurse checked Lilli's vitals and another nurse drew 13 vials of blood, Lilli had to go to various floors of the clinic for additional tests. This brought back memories of all that we had endured the previous year. As someone who never served in the military, I couldn't say that it felt like going back to a battlefield, but I felt like I was going back to the site of trauma. I couldn't imagine how the doctors, nurses, and staff managed to endure this ongoing trauma of life and death, but I was thankful for this team of people who were called to serve our daughter in spite of all the negative and scary aspects of pediatric oncology.

While we waited for various tests in waiting rooms spread out from one floor to another of the clinic, Lilli bumped into a few kids who had been on the unit at the same time as her. What a relief to see some of the other patients out of the hospital, surviving, and to some degree thriving. These survivors posed for photos and compared notes about their post-transplant recovery processes.

Lilli repeated the echocardiogram, x-rays, pulmonary functioning tests, blood tests, and a bone density test, a new test for us. With all the blood that was drawn from her body, Lilli was light-headed until we could grab a bite for lunch. Unlike the previous year, Lilli had been cleared to be in public places, and she walked with me and LouAnne down to the food court. While we waited to be called back to an exam room, Lilli caught up with Josh, who was excited to show off pictures of his newborn baby. Lilli was shy but happy to share some of her plans for high school in the coming year and to show off her sock design. There were long lines for food and long lines for labs and long lines at the check-in counters for all these tests. It turned into a full day of studies and waiting for studies before we could make it back to the transplant clinic to meet with Dr. Martin and Erika, the Pediatric Nurse Practitioner.

After reviewing Lilli's initial labs and test results on the computer, Dr. Martin gave Lilli some good news that she had been waiting over a year to hear. He finally gave her permission to eat a fresh salad with fresh fruits and vegetables again. Lilli was ecstatic. Most kids might've missed cheeseburgers. Lilli missed fresh fruits and vegetables. For balance, though, Lilli was also given permission to eat desserts from bakeries and doughnut shops again. Lilli realized that she'd finally be able to eat doughnuts from our favorite local place, and it was like Christmas morning. Dr. Martin reduced Lilli's medication list slightly, examined Lilli, said how great she looked for one year post-transplant, and said that she didn't have to come back for another year.

A week later, we got an email from the team at Duke informing us that Lilli's chimerism labs turned out great. There was still no trace of Lilli's old DNA in any of the blood samples, and Donor #2 was still winning the long-term battle for control of Lilli's bone marrow and blood production. I gave out a sigh of relief and shed a tear over the good news. At one year post-transplant, Lilli appeared to be in such good health that she might be one of those 85% of patients who survive the transplant process and continue to live.

Whew! What a relief to hear that the donor cells are still winning out. I don't want to jinx it, but it seems like Lilli's old DNA is completely gone from her blood. If she becomes a criminal someday, then they won't be able to pin her down from blood evidence alone. Ha!

Dr. Martin gave Lilli permission to return to the classroom, and she was ecstatic. She went back in time to wrap up 8th grade at Brown Summit Middle, where she had attended half of 6th grade, half of 7th grade, and almost none of 8th grade in person. She had been a virtual student in a school full of high achieving scholars. At one point in 6th grade, Lilli had shown interest in applying for some of the magnet high school options, options that would've continued her trajectory through advanced or specialized schools. After all that she endured in middle school, however, Lilli was determined to be normal in high school and to attend our neighborhood school. She didn't apply to other high schools, but she did apply for the special IB, or International Baccalaureate, program in our neighborhood school, Grimsley.

At the end of 8th grade, Lilli's school hosted its traditional end-of-year awards ceremony. This was familiar territory for us. I was an emotional wreck during Lilli's 6th grade ceremony. We missed her 7th grade ceremony because we were living in the transplant unit of the hospital. Lilli returned to school just in time to attend the 8th grade ceremony, in which she and a small group of friends performed Anna Kendrick's version of "When I'm Gone," or "Cups." I was certain they chose this song to make grown men cry, but I was determined to keep my emotions in check that day. Two years earlier, I sat in the front row to shield myself from people's glances. That morning I decided to sit right in the middle of this group of parents, grandparents, and other family members.

Lilli was recognized for having straight As for the year and for having straight As all three years of middle school. She was among a large group of students who had maintained that level of academic excellence for their entire tenure at the school, and Principal Mott took the privilege of calling out the names of these students. Just before she announced Lilli's name, Ms. Mott described all the things that Lilli had gone through during middle school and how special it was that Lilli had maintained her grades in spite of all her hardships. She said, "This student deserves some special recognition because she fought cancer multiple times and had a bone marrow transplant. She was isolated and had to finish middle school from home. I'm proud that she has achieved all As for all three years at Brown Summit...Lilli Hicks."

When Ms. Mott called out Lilli's name, I jumped up to give Lilli a standing ovation. I had not planned on this public display, in the same way that I had not planned on bawling my eyes out two years earlier, but I did it. I looked around to see the entire gym full of students and guests also standing up to cheer on Lilli and to celebrate her life as much as her academics. The woman seated next to me, a stranger to me before our brief conversation about faith and life as we waited for the ceremony to begin, said, "I thought there was something special about you. Now I see. That's your daughter, isn't it?" I nodded.

I looked at LouAnne on my other side, and we both swelled with pride and emotions. No tears flowed that day, at least none of mine flowed in public. We stayed after the ceremony for the annual cookout at the school, and I tried to blend in like all the other parents of normal kids, students who just so happened to be some of the brightest kids in the county. Over hamburgers and hotdogs, LouAnne and I connected with a mom, a runner whom I followed on Strava but had not met in person. Lilli blended right in with the crowd. She played games. She talked to her friends. She laughed. She changed into her BSMS Alumni t-shirt and enjoyed the cookout. It was a beautiful sight.

Fully Crazy

After running a few half marathons and planning to run a few more, I decided to sign up for a full marathon. I searched for marathons close enough to home that I wouldn't have to travel far and wouldn't have to train for a totally different terrain or elevation. I discovered the RDC Marathon that was announcing its inaugural marathon in the fall of 2017. This marathon, organized to raise funds for ALS research at Duke, hit home. Not only was I a fan of Duke Health but I was also employed at one time by Phil Freelon, the most well-known African-American architect, who had recently been diagnosed with ALS, a debilitating disease with no cure.

I registered for the full marathon, and then the organizers announced a competition to design the race medals. I had to enter. Influenced by the background story for the race, based on a former ALS patient who got tattoos of black swallows, I designed a medal with prominent swallows encircling runners of different ability levels, including a runner on a recumbent bike, inspired by Andrea, a marathoner battling ALS. The piece-de-resistance of my design was the idea for a silhouette cutout of a swallow that would give each medal-earner the chance to create a swallow *light tattoo* by positioning the medal in relation to sunlight and one's body. I won the design competition, which came with a prize of a free registration for the marathon.

I have to run this marathon now. I mean, how many people can say that they designed the medal for their first marathon? I will be in that small number after this race.

I trained for months, following a generic training plan that I found in a Runner's World magazine. It marked the first time I followed any kind of plan, and I managed to hit most of the training paces, distances, and runs per week. Training was like having a second job, and it tested my family's patience. "Can't you talk about something other than running?" LouAnne said, "and you're always tired on Saturdays after your long runs. I need you to help more around the house." I was inspired to run because I wanted to be there for my family, but running had also taken me away from my family. Finding balance in my running remained a struggle.

Lilli and Amelia rode with me to Durham two nights before the race, to the Durham Bulls Athletic Park, to pick up my race packet, t-shirt, sweatshirt, and racing bib. "This is your first marathon?" said the volunteer, "then you're bound to have a PR."

"Yes, I guess that's one way to look at it," I replied.

The girls and I saw sample medals on a display table, the first time I saw my medal design realized. The full marathon and half marathon medals were based on my design, and the 5k was smaller and based on a different design. Seeing the medals provided the final bit of motivation to run a strong race. Heading out of the race expo we bumped into a few former co-workers, including a friend who had taken up running marathons a few years before I did. "Pace yourself, and you'll do fine," he said, "I do one marathon a year, and it's a fun challenge to train for them."

Saturday night before the race I drove back to Durham and had dinner with a different former co-worker at PF Chang's where I could get my fill of carbs from the stir-fried rice. I stayed at a hotel close to the Streets of Southpoint Mall in Durham, where the race would begin, and I awoke bright and early to run my very first marathon. I had laid out my running clothes in the hotel room the night before the race, and I had packed Vaseline, instead of talcum powder and large round band-aids, for those chafe-prone areas on my body (I have since graduated to Body Glide and Aquaphor). I stashed plenty of energy gels in my water bottle wrapper, and I ate a light breakfast of a banana, half a bagel, and coconut water.

I was as nervous at that starting line as I was for my first 5k at the high school track near Charlotte. When the race started it was around 29 degrees Fahrenheit, and it didn't warm up much throughout the race. I had dreamed of running a sub-4:00 marathon. Much like breaking 100 in golf, it's the average person's dream goal. While the world class marathoners run fast and can finish in around two hours, I was dreaming of being half as fast (or is it twice as slow?) and running 3:59:59 or faster. I started out the race a little faster than I had anticipated, a common mistake for even experienced runners, but then I got into a groove of an easy pace for miles and miles. At one point, I was on the heels of the 4:00 pacing group.

I feel great, and I can run a little faster than the 4:00 group. Maybe I'll speed up and work towards the next pacing group.

My mind was playing tricks on me in part because the race had a simultaneous start for half marathoners and full marathoners. I was running mostly with half marathoners who had to sustain their pace for half the distance, and I got sucked into the foolish notion that I could maintain that pace for the entire marathon.

Just before the halfway point I passed the 3:45 pacing group. I should've known better, but I felt like I was on top of the world and was poised to obliterate my goal of 3:59:59. But once the half marathoners peeled off and I found myself alone on a trail of rolling hills for as far as the eye could see, I realized the error in my judgment. I started slowing down around miles 19-20, and by mile 21 I was walking-running-walking-running and eating a big slice of humble pie. I watched as the 3:45 pacing group passed me around mile 22. Ouch! And then I watched as the 4:00 pacing group passed me around mile 24. How demoralizing! I started doing the math, based on my GARMIN running watch, to figure out my best and worst-case scenarios. 3:59 was out of the question. 4:05 was about the best I could hope for, and I thought 4:15 was my worst-case. I found enough energy to run the last ¼ mile, and I finished in 4:09:05 officially. I should've felt great to have finished my first full marathon and to have been within 20 seconds/mile of my goal pace, but I let my dream goal steal my joy.

I became determined to run another marathon as quickly as possible and started eyeing a spring 2018 marathon, but fate would have other plans for me. The RDC was in early November 2017, and I took it easy for a few weeks following that race. I did not, however, follow the textbook advice of taking it easy for 26 days following 26.2 miles of a marathon. When December rolled around, I was back to running 5-10-mile runs by the time of Lilli's cancer-versary. She was initially diagnosed on December 13, 2014, 12/13/14, and the previous year I started a tradition of running 12.13 miles on December 13. On December 13, 2017, I left the house, drove to Country Park—my normal running route—and set out to run my 12.13 miles. In the first mile or two I felt some pain in my left ankle. I had been feeling that pain for a few days, but I had ignored it. I figured, "What's the worst that could happen? I'll get over a sore ankle in a few days. Maybe running on it will help it warm up, and it won't be a big deal." Boy, was I ever wrong. I was in pain for most of the 12.13 miles, and the pain didn't stop when I finished running.

After running pain-free and injury-free for two years, I had sustained my first running injury. It was entirely self-inflicted, as I failed to listen to my body. I felt indestructible and like my 40-something-year-old body would bounce back the same way it did when I was a teenager and had a sprained ankle. I struggled to walk down steps. I struggled to do calf raises or to stretch my left foot. I read all I could online to diagnose myself, and I concluded that I had a textbook case of PTTD, or Posterior Tibial Tendon Dysfunction. To add insult to injury, I read that PTTD is a disorder mostly experienced by middle-aged (check), obese (not anymore), women (not at all). I had avoided all the normal running injuries only to succumb to an injury that was uncommon among my demographic.

PTTD treatment included the Rest-Ice-Compression-Elevation (RICE) method, some strengthening exercises, and time. After a few weeks of not running at all and still feeling some pain, I went to see an orthopedist at the same clinic that had helped with my ruptured disc seven years earlier. The doctor diagnosed me with flat feet and a mild case of PTTD. He prescribed taking it easy and slowly easing back into my mileage and pace. He also suggested that if the pain persisted I should come back and talk to his colleague who was better with feet. Lastly, he said that I should have my running shoes re-evaluated.

The dream of a second marathon within six months of my first one went out the window. I could barely run 2-3 miles, and I was in pain every time I ran. I took some inspiration from having watched Lilli go through her chemotherapy treatments and stem cell transplant, and I figured that I was at my low point like Lilli experienced during each month of chemo and during her transplant. I would have to wait until my body recovered. In my case it was a recovery of a tendon and the neighboring muscles, not my bone marrow and blood cells. While Lilli's body recovered after 2-3 weeks, I was looking at 2-3 months from what I read about PTTD.

I tried the RICE method. I tried stretching. I tried ankle braces. I tried changing my running shoes (I had suspected that my running shoe change shortly before my injury had contributed to the injury). I tried using KT tape on my left ankle for each and every run. Some of these techniques were easier and cheaper to maintain than others, and I continued taping my ankle and wearing a better fitting running shoe. In time, I was able to get over my injury, and I regained the distance and pace of my running after months of nursing my injury.

Early Birthday Presents

Lilli's middle school, which had become Amelia's middle school, had roughly 250 students. Lilli went from that tiny school to Grimsley High School with nearly 1,800 students, over 400 students per grade. Lilli had one main goal for 9th grade: to have a normal school year. She desperately wanted to blend in and to have no more medical emergencies or complications to disrupt her life. Ninth grade fulfilled Lilli's dreams of normalcy. She continued playing violin and joined the high school orchestra. She joined the Battle-of-the-Books team for avid readers. She went to high school football games. She hung out with friends. She was able to attend Girl Scout meetings in person. Except for the regular check-ups with her oncologists, Lilli had an average school year, finishing with straight As and near the top of her class.

Lilli worked on her Girl Scout Silver Award project that year. She joined forces with another scout from our church to give back to the Ronald McDonald House (RMH) that had become our home away from home. Lilli and her friend planned a sustainable system to collect pop tabs at our church and to turn them in to the RMH. The RMH collects these pop tabs, found on soda cans, tennis ball cans, dog food cans, vegetable cans, and other cans, and sells them to scrap metal recyclers to pay the electric bills for the facility. While we couldn't give back to the RMH financially, as we still had thousands of dollars in debt and ongoing annual medical bills, we could mobilize our church friends, neighbors, and family members to collect pop tabs. We delivered over 100 pounds of pop tabs that first year.

In June of 2018, Lilli had her annual check-up at Duke, including all the same tests, labs, and waiting around in the clinic and hospital as the previous year's check-up. The team was impressed by how well Lilli looked and how far she had come in two years. I didn't worry at all as Lilli and I left the Duke hospital campus and drove back to Greensboro.

About a week after Lilli's check-up, I drove the family home from vacation bible school one evening. We had been living high on life, not a care in the world compared to two years before that. After we pulled into the driveway, the rest of the family went inside the house while I stayed outside to check out the flower bed beside our driveway and in front of our porch. The daylilies were in full bloom, and I was thinking about how nice it was to have the freedom to think about the plants in our yard again when my phone rang. I pulled it out of my front left pocket to see that it was a 919 area code number from the Triangle. "Mr. Hicks, this is Paul Martin."

WHAT?! I've heard this kind of phone call before.

Oncologists don't call me out of the blue on a summer evening to chat about the weather or to deliver excellent news about Lilli. "There's nothing to worry about, but I wanted to let you know something about Lilli's latest chimerism results over the phone so that you're not surprised when you see it posted online or in the letter that we send to Dr. Buckley." Dr. Martin proceeded to tell me that while the chimerism (amount of donor cells vs. Lilli's old cells) tests still showed that there were greater than 98% donor cells, the tests revealed a *trace* of Lilli's old DNA. Of the three different results, two of the three results showed no trace. Only the myeloid fraction of the blood came back with a trace of Lilli's old DNA. After absorbing the initial shock of this news, I realized that the trace was found in the same type of blood cells that initially mutated into cancerous cells. Dr. Martin didn't say that out loud, but I could make my own connections.

While Dr. Martin tried to reassure me that the team at Duke wasn't overly concerned about these results, he couldn't stop my mind from jumping to the worst-case scenario: that Lilli's old cancerous cells had been hanging out for two years just waiting to pounce. He said that we shouldn't be worried, either, but that he wanted Lilli to have her blood checked again three months later. He added that when the results first showed up he doubted their accuracy and

361

asked that the lab re-test the sample, which they did. When they rechecked the sample, they came up with the same results.

I stood outside the minivan, alone in the driveway, with just the late afternoon worn-out daylily blooms to keep me company as I tried to compose myself. I asked what the possible outcomes and scenarios could be. Dr. Martin said that if there were still a trace in three months that they would check again at Lilli's three-year post-transplant. He said that if there were no trace in three months (there had been no trace of Lilli's old DNA at every previous chimerism test), then they also would test again at the next annual check-up. I asked what if the trace were to become a larger percentage in time, and he said that they would conduct additional tests if that were the case. While I didn't press him on what these tests would be, I assumed that there would be more bone marrow tests and blood tests to see what kinds of cells were present and to check for any new cancerous cells. He said that if we had any more questions about this news to give him a call.

I was on the phone when LouAnne looked out the side door from the kitchen, noticing the concern on my face. She came out while I was still on the phone and heard the end of my conversation with Dr. Martin.

"Who was that, Travis? Should we be worried?" LouAnne asked.

I explained what Dr. Martin shared with me, and LouAnne and I agreed that we should call Lilli outside to tell her the news. LouAnne walked back up the three steps to the kitchen door and said, "Lilli! Come outside. We have something to tell you." Dappled late afternoon sunlight washed across Lilli's face as she opened the door and looked at me quizzically.

"There's some news, Lilli…nothing to worry about, that Dr. Martin just shared with me over the phone. Why don't we call him right back?" I suggested.

I put the phone on speaker and asked Dr. Martin to repeat what he had told me. Lilli looked a little startled to hear the news but was not emotional nor upset about it, since Dr. Martin reassured us that the team there was not worried about the results. After a few moments of silent head nods, Lilli went back inside while LouAnne and I stood in the driveway, shocked to hear this news after such great progress Lilli had made over the first two years post-transplant.

"Are you worried?" LouAnne asked.

"I can't stop shaking," I said, "I feel like I did the first night we were told to go to the emergency room." I shook uncontrollably and stood in the driveway until I got my body back under control. I couldn't go inside and let the kids see me in that condition. LouAnne put her arms around me and held on tight until I calmed down.

I can't tell LouAnne how worried I am, but I'm worried! Lilli could accomplish great things in her life. She could run 20 marathons. She could save a million lives. She could become the fifth female President of the United States. Despite all of this, though, I'll live in fear that she is but a split second or one more lab result from going right back into a life-and-death situation.

It was early summer, and the thought crossed my mind that it might be our final summer as a family of five. The clock was ticking down from three months until they would re-test Lilli's blood for the percentage of donor cells. For a day or two I was feeling low, imagining the worst outcome possible. I finally talked myself out of this self-pity and decided to do my best to make the summer as special and memorable as possible, within our modest means, and to enjoy every day as it presented itself. As there was no 100% guarantee that any one of our family members would live through the summer, I decided that I'd not let the fear of *"what if"* rule my attitude all summer.

I announced to all the kids that they'd get their birthday presents two months early, as soon as I got my paycheck at the end of June. I was teaching a summer studio as I had for several years, and teaching summer courses meant extra pay during the summer. My paycheck at the end of June would be my largest of the year, and I decided that we'd take some of that extra salary and put it towards these early birthday presents (all three kids were born in September). Lilli wanted a new bicycle, as she hadn't had a bike her size in years. Amelia wanted a new guitar, as she had been playing LouAnne's old guitar, the one I got her for our five-year wedding anniversary (the same day my mom passed away), which was a) not her own, and b) a classical nylon string guitar and not the six string she wanted to be playing. And Collin wanted a subscription to Xbox online so that he could play more games on his Xbox. The one thought that I couldn't bear to share with the kids was this, "if this is going to be Lilli's last summer with us, then I'd like to see her enjoy the new bike that she's dreamed about. And I'd like to see her brother and sister enjoy their birthday presents early, too."

When September came and it was time for Lilli's blood to be checked once more, I took Lilli to Brenner like it was a normal monthly check-up. We walked in to the clinic, checked in with the receptionist, had Lilli's vitals checked, and then went to Miss Pat's blood draw lab. Pat drew Lilli's blood, filled all the vials required for the normal labs plus the chimerism labs to be sent off to the lab across the country. We then went out to wait in the waiting room where Lilli was called back to see Dr. Buckley for her regular check-up. The normal lab results were back quickly that day, and Lilli's blood looked great. We would have to wait a week or two for the chimerism results to know if Lilli's old DNA had grown in proportion or not.

The following week I was teaching my fall semester design studio when I got a text from LouAnne telling me that new lab results had been posted on DukeMyChart, the online interface for labs, appointments, other test results, and messages from Lilli's team. LouAnne couldn't remember the password and asked me to check the results. I had to excuse myself from class to check this message, in case I were to find out devastating news. When I logged in to the website, I saw that the new results appeared; however, when I clicked on the link to the results, I found a "yes" under the lab results section, but that was it. No more details were posted…just a "yes," meaning that there were lab results, but they weren't posted.

My heart was pounding through my chest as I headed down to the faculty mailroom to find some privacy and reach out to Dr. Martin at Duke. I e-mailed him to ask, "I see that there are new lab results posted online. Is there anything that we need to talk about?" After sending that e-mail I waited for a few tense minutes, wondering how the response would go. Would we be heading to Duke for additional tests and to talk about the next steps in Lilli's battle with leukemia? Or would I be able to breathe again after holding my breath for the past three months? The air was sucked out of the room while I awaited a response.

It didn't take long for Dr. Martin to respond to my e-mail, and it was a quick and to-the-point response, "Labs are excellent. No trace of Lilli's old DNA. See you at next year's annual check-up." I couldn't believe our good fortune and couldn't wait to share it with LouAnne and Lilli. I texted both of them right away, as LouAnne was at work and Lilli was in class at her new high school. "Tears of joy," I said, "No trace of Lilli's old DNA." I could breathe again, for the first time in three months since that phone call in the driveway. This experience would be our new normal each year following Lilli's annual check-up.

My life as a pediatric cancer father involves all kinds of stress leading up to check-ups, not knowing how the check-up will go, how the lab results will go, and how the follow-up phone call will go. This will be my life from here on out. I will worry about Lilli, but I'll try to balance my worry with faith...and an attempt to live in the moment and not become too anxious about the future. Each day of the journey has been a blessing, and I wouldn't wish to have forgone the journey by jumping to today.

Three-Year Post

My experience the previous year of getting that phone call as I sat in our driveway still haunted me. On the best of days, I did not think one bit about the possibility of Lilli's old cells returning. On the worst of days, I interpreted every yawn, cough, sneeze, or bug bite as some sign of cancer. I tried to live somewhere between optimism and the reality of our past experiences, but the return trip to Durham and Duke brought my anxiety and paranoia to the surface. If Lilli's old cells were in the process of returning, I didn't want to know it; however, if the donor's cells were still winning, I would've welcomed that news. From previous experience, I knew that it would take a week or so to find out those chimerism results. I knew that I would worry until getting the news from the lab. I did my best to shield my feelings from Lilli and pretend like her three-year post-transplant appointment would be a walk in the park.

Lilli's check-up that Monday morning in June of 2019 turned out to be the fastest visit we ever had to the hospital. LouAnne asked me to take Lilli for the appointment so she could teach her preschool music classes that morning, and I obliged. Following an uneventful hour-long drive to Durham, Lilli and I parked on our favorite basement level of the parking deck and walked across Erwin Road to the Children's Health Center. Walking into the light-filled lobby and atrium, Lilli suggested we take the stairs. "These steps aren't as steep as the stairs at my school, and we won't have to wait on the elevator," Lilli said. We walked up to the fourth floor and checked in.

We sat in the waiting area for a brief time, commenting on how quiet the waiting area was for a Monday morning. With such a light patient load that morning, the nurse called Lilli for her vitals check in record time. After vitals, we returned to the waiting area to wait again. Our chairs didn't even have a chance to warm up before we heard, "Lillian Hicks." It seemed like we were on record pace for that clinic.

We walked back to the small room where Lilli took a seat and prepared to have her blood drawn. I took my normal position standing near the door, a nervous Dad with an aversion to the sight of blood. The nurse filled seven vials of blood, about half the amount they typically drew. Lilli reminded me that in previous years the team drew extra blood to be submitted for a research study led by Dr. Martin that had wrapped up. "Do you need some juice or a Coke, Lilli?" I asked.

"No, I'm fine," she said, and we left for the next appointment.

At that point, we were about 45 minutes ahead of schedule for our next appointment with the echocardiogram technician, but I said, "Let's just go ahead and check in to see what happens." Lilli and I walked back down the stairs to the ground floor lobby, checked in at the large reception desk, sat down in an area off to ourselves, and waited to be called back for the echo. I finally had a chance to survey the surroundings while sitting down for a minute. The lobby and atrium hadn't changed much, if at all, since the last time we were there. The same green and orange feathery mobiles flitted around in mid-air, filling the high volume of space, and the same aquarium anchored the colorful glass-sided elevators that carried sick kids up and down. Fully prepared to wait 45 minutes, I was surprised to hear Lilli's name called five minutes later.

A technician escorted us into the restricted corridor to one of the echo rooms. Lilli changed into a gown and decided to watch some TV for old time's sake. While living together in various hospital rooms, Lilli and I had compiled a short list of favorite channels and TV shows. That morning we decided to watch some HGTV to kill time. We didn't even make it through a half hour episode before the echo was finished and Lilli could move on to the chest x-ray down the hall. Lilli was smart enough not to wear any metal that day, which made the x-ray go quickly. By the time Lilli finished with the x-ray, we were an hour ahead of schedule.

Trying our luck once more, I suggested that we go ahead and report to the second floor for a PFT, or Pulmonary Functioning Test. I pointed out to the staff that we were an hour early but asked if they could work in Lilli ahead of schedule. The receptionist said, "I think we just called her name. Let's see." Lilli and I sat down in the waiting area and were called back immediately. After finishing the strenuous PFT, Lilli was thirsty. I couldn't blame her, given all she had to do to blow in and out of this machine for the better part of 20 minutes.

We took the stairs from the second floor down to the main level and walked down the long corridor between the Children's Health Center and the main hospital. We turned the corner and walked past the adult radiology waiting area to the hub of circulation where the spokes from the children's center, emergency department, and elevator lobby intersected. We crossed paths with people coming in from the main entry lobby, folks going to the adult cancer center, and people coming and going from the cafeteria, Subway, and Starbucks. Lilli and I stopped by the Starbucks for drinks since we had plenty of time to spare. We returned to the 4th floor around 11:00, hoping that there might be a chance for us to get in to see Dr. Martin before lunchtime.

We barely waited before heading back to an exam room. Lauren, one of the Nurse Practitioners, knocked on the door after a few minutes. She looked at Lilli and commented on how great she looked. She went over Lilli's med list, her recent history, and her preliminary labs. The PFT results were in, and they all looked good. The CBC and metabolic labs were also in, and they all looked perfectly normal according to Lauren. Lilli pointed out a rash that was on her trunk, a rash that appeared a day before Lilli headed home from Florida where she, Amelia, and others from the church youth group had gone to work on hurricane-damaged homes. Lilli had come back with what appeared to be a heat rash, and Lauren wasn't too concerned about the rash. The night before Lilli's appointment, LouAnne had whispered the word "leukemia" as it can sometimes present itself as a rash. I was relieved to hear Lauren say that she thought it was a heat rash.

Lauren remarked to Lilli, "Is this your natural hair? It's been growing out long enough since you were taking cyclosporine that it's not cyclosporine hair. But it wasn't curly before your transplant? No? Well, it's beautiful hair."

I always thought that somehow my family genes with curly, wavy, and thick hair had something to do with Lilli's hair growing back a little curly. I said, "No, Lilli's hair was straight and thick before transplant, but now it's so curly that she will straighten it sometimes for a change."

Dr. Martin knocked on the door and was all smiles. He remarked on how well Lilli looked and took a look at her trunk and the rash. He said that it could also be bed bugs if not a heat rash. He asked Lilli about how and where she slept while in Florida, and he said, "It sounds like it could be bed bugs if it doesn't get better soon." Dr. Martin talked to us about stretching out Lilli's appointments to 6 months with Brenner and still annually with him. We also talked about transitioning from pediatrics to adult care. He said that the adult cancer center at Duke has a late-effects clinic that is world class and that he would highly recommend it for Lilli.

I guess I should brace myself for the adult Lilli. In two years Lilli will be going off to college and won't be under our roof full-time. I'm gonna have a hard time with that one.

"Lilli, can you believe we made it out of the clinic in such record time? I feel great!" I said. It was the shortest annual check-up Lilli ever had. We finished before lunchtime, and Lilli chose PDQ, one of her favorite fast food places that we didn't have in Greensboro. We returned to Greensboro after lunch, and LouAnne couldn't believe how early we had returned home. While I wanted to enjoy the day and the quick clinic visit, the fear of Lilli's chimerism results weighed heavily on my mind.

The first day after Lilli's appointment was too soon for us to expect any results from the chimerism labs, and we didn't hear anything from the team. The following day, a Wednesday, was still most likely too soon, and we heard nothing. Just in case we were going to hear early results, however, I logged into LouAnne's e-mail on my phone. Lilli's transplant team had my phone number for texting and LouAnne's e-mail address for e-mail messages. There was no e-mail message that day.

The longer it took for us to hear Lilli's chimerism results, the more nervous I got. When the previous year's labs revealed a trace of Lilli's old DNA, the transplant team asked the lab to re-run the labs to see if there was some mistake. Was it going to be the same this year? Thursday morning, I checked LouAnne's e-mail again. I scrolled down a few lines and found that the team had just e-mailed LouAnne with a brief note. Getting an e-mail was the first good sign. Bad news would come from a phone call, but good news would come in an e-mail. I opened the e-mail to find out that there was no trace of Lilli's old DNA. Hallelujah! I couldn't wait to tell LouAnne. I ran from the bedroom to the living room to check in with LouAnne. She had just seen the message, too, and we shared a brief moment together to celebrate the good news. Then I yelled to Lilli who was in her bed, "Lilli, it's all donor cells. None of your old DNA! Great news, LilliBoo!"

I can breathe again, at least until Lilli's next clinic appointment. Such is the life of a pediatric cancer father.

And now I'm about to head out for a 10-mile run as I train for my fifth marathon in 2.5 years. Such is the life of a long-distance runner.

Acknowledgements

Throughout the journey of writing this book I received encouragement and advice from a lot of people, mostly friends and family as well as acquaintances through Facebook and Instagram. I found a supportive online community who kept me going with this book when I found myself struggling to relive all these experiences and to recall details that were painful and scary the first time around and difficult to relive the second time around. I'd like to thank those people who read excerpts from the book and provided encouragement and criticism, and I'd like to thank my family for tolerating my newfound interest in writing and the time that this project has taken away from our family time. I hope that you all can find something meaningful from this book in time.

The doctors, nurses, nursing assistants, therapists, and other hospital staff were amazing in their abilities to care for Lilli. Some of them became like members of our family for the time we spent in the hospital. While I won't recall all of their names, here are the names of some of the folks who kept our daughter alive and well: O'Kelley, Wofford, McLean, Buckley, Russell, Dixon, Castellino, Martin, Prasad, Driscoll, Page, McAlister, Larrier, Erika, Kat, Lauren, Diane, Jane, Nancy, Mary, Laura, Marcia, Kim, Teirraha, Liz, Danny, Jo, Pat, Leslie, Jennifer, the other Jennifer, the other-other Jennifer, Julie, Jessica, Loren, Rachel, the other Rachel, Catherine, Katie, Liz, Alyssa, Angela, Brittany, Ashley, Jess, Angela, Kirbie, Leslie, Stacy, the other Stacy, the other-other Stacy, Tracy, the other Tracy, Colin, Marty, Shelby, Robyn, Lindsay, Michelle, Whitney, Linda, Maria, Marion, Jill, Jenna, Christina, Bobbie, Jamie, Paige, Shelby, Josh, Hillary, Caroline, Jeff, Linda, Ruth, Darlene, Trey, Connie, and Joan. It's sad that any child has to go through cancer treatments, but I'm grateful for people like these who have answered a calling to care for pediatric cancer patients.

There's no way that LouAnne and I could've maintained our sanity and our family without the help of our extended family. LouAnne's parents, Joe and Janet Watson, dropped everything they were doing to move 340 miles away from home and move into our basement for months at a time. My father, Lee Hicks, provided moral and financial support along the way. My aunt, Teresa, and sister, Tammy, took some of the stress off my in-laws by spending weeks with us along the way. Other family members who spent time with us in the hospital or at home during this time included Sidney, Toni, Teri, Danny, Wayne, Kirk, Jennifer, Tyler, Lydia, Lauren, Bruce, Barbara, and Richard. Other family members from the Hicks, Watson, and Dominy families also came through for us. We couldn't have made it without your support.

Our community came through with all kinds of support along the way, and I'm bound to forget some of the names of people who helped carry our burdens. Those people were from our church families at Guilford College United Methodist Church, Greenwood Forest Baptist Church, Louisburg Baptist Church, Northside Baptist Church, Philadelphia United Methodist Church, and Wesley Chapel United Methodist Church. We also got support from our Greensboro community in Westwood, General Greene Elementary School, and Brown Summit Middle School. Kisses 4 Kate, Resilience Gives, Family Reach, and Make-A-Wish came through with emotional and financial support, and the Ronald McDonald House of Durham & Wake became our home away from home. Childhood friends from Putnam County and Baldwin County, Georgia, delivered on fundraisers and other financial and emotional support. And our college friends and campus ministers from Georgia Tech, Princeton, and Georgia College were there for us when we called on them. Former co-workers and students from New Jersey, the Triangle Area of North Carolina, NC State University, and UNC Greensboro came through for us, too. We needed all the support we could get, and we got a lot of support from friends, family, neighbors, colleagues, acquaintances, and perfect strangers.

As I compiled all my ideas into this manuscript, I got help from people who really knew what they were doing, like beta readers, Jeannine, Pat, Christina, Marshall, Steffi, Kathie, Buck, and Scott; Jennifer from the UNCG Writing Center; and Barbara, who proofread the book.

If you ever have to go through a life-threatening illness, then I pray that you have the support that we have felt through our journey.

And if you decide to write about your life experiences, then I pray that you find a group of people as supportive as I have. Peace be with you and yours.

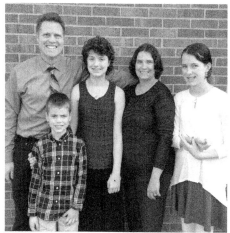
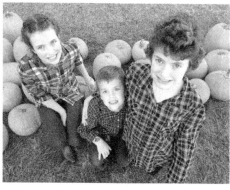
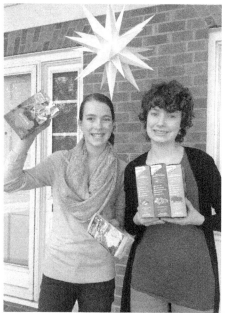
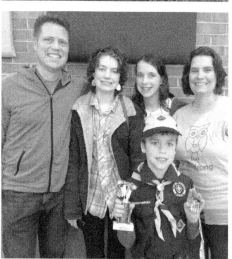
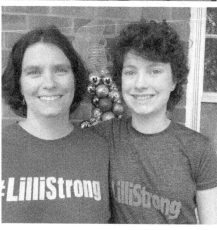
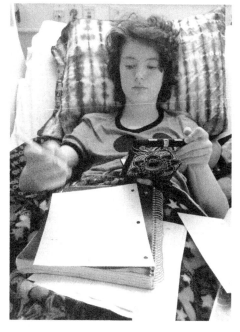

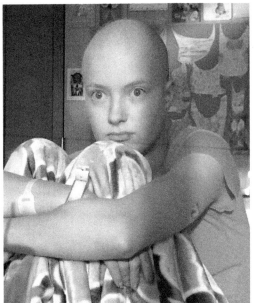
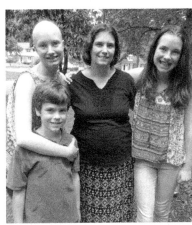
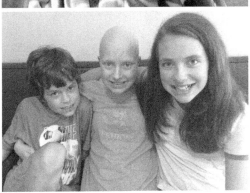
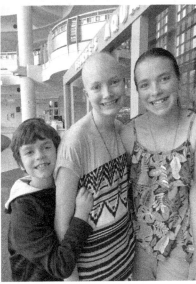
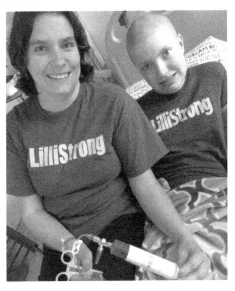
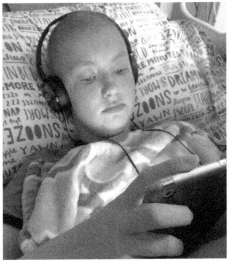

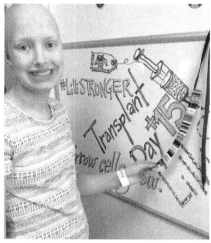
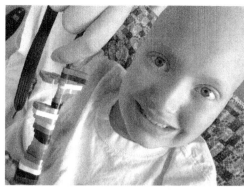
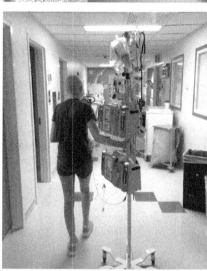
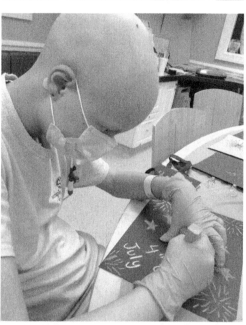
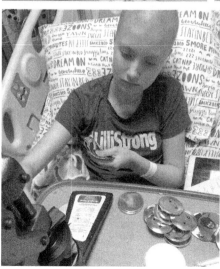
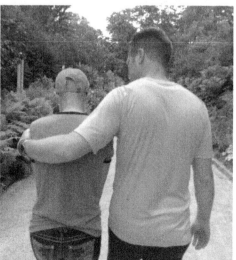

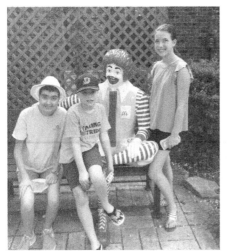
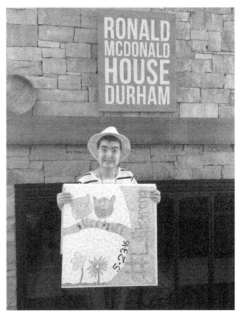
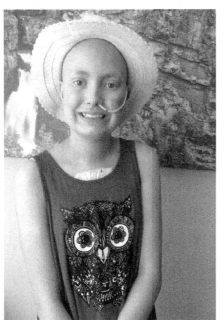
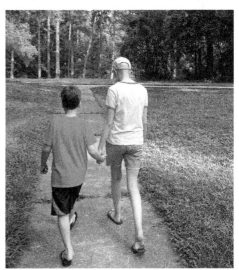
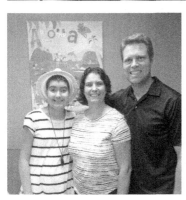
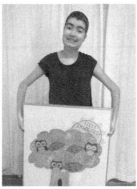
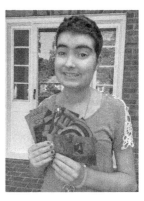

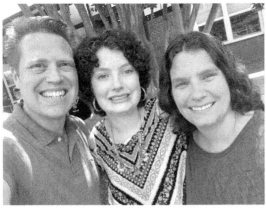
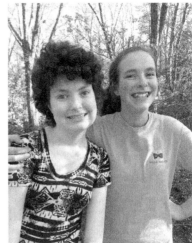
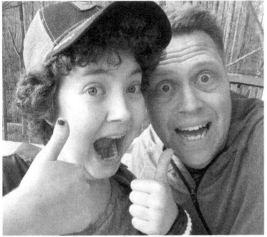
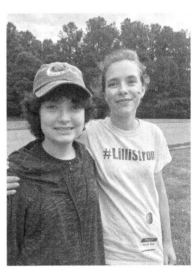
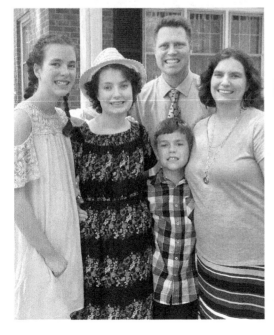
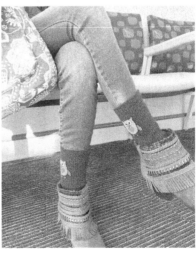

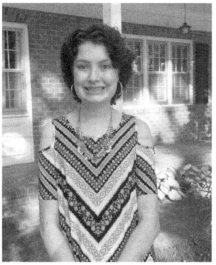
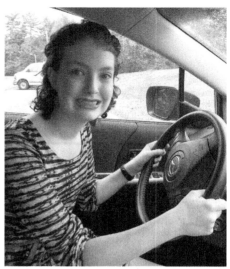
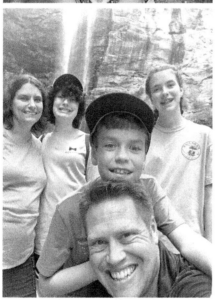
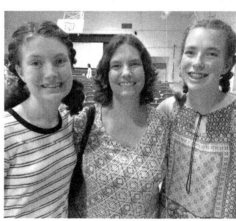
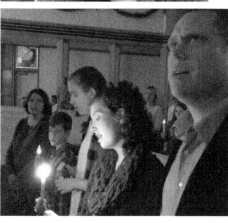
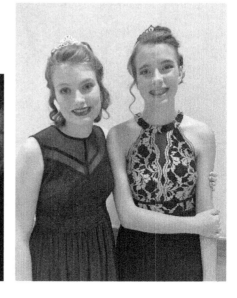

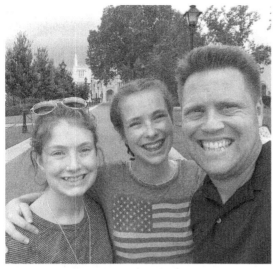
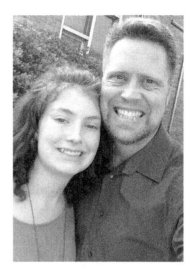
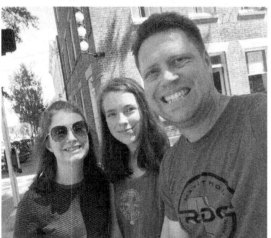
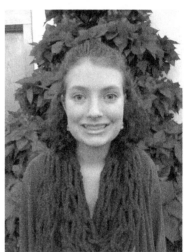
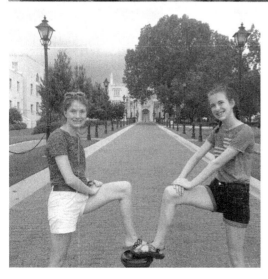
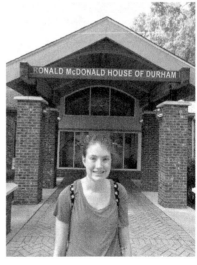

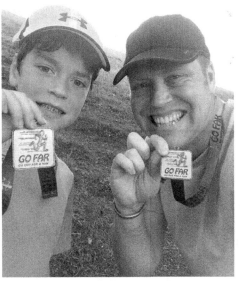
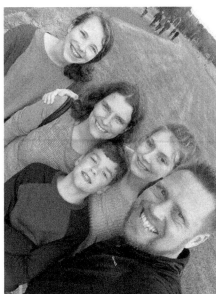
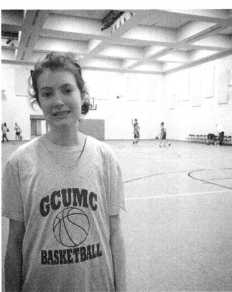
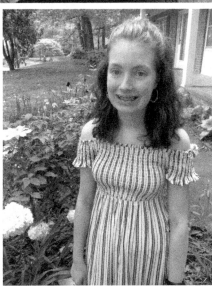
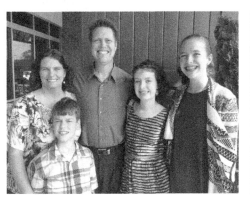
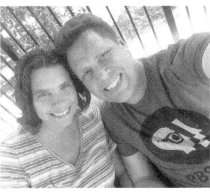

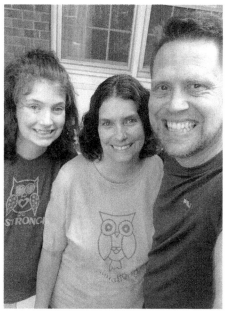

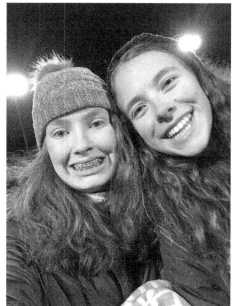

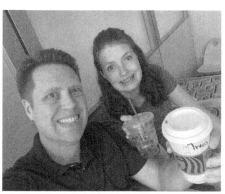

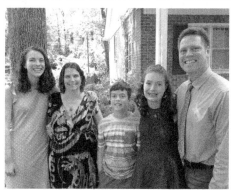

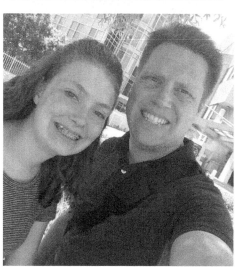

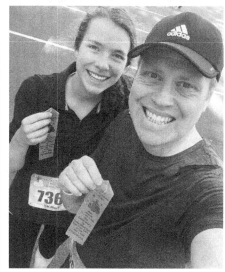

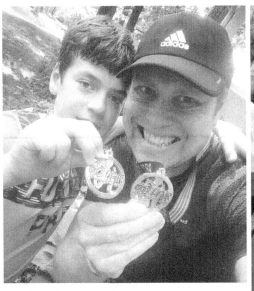
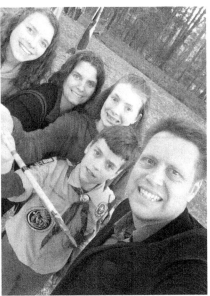
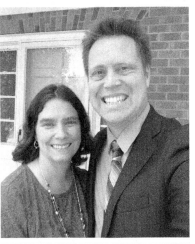
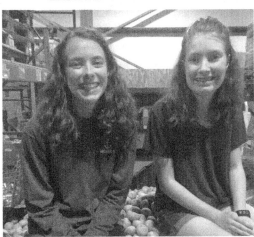
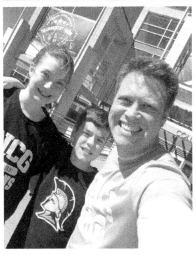
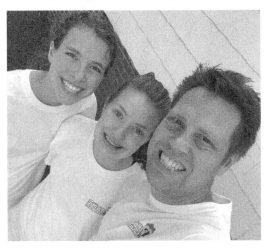

For Discussion

1. The Hicks family relied on their community in the midst of medical crises. **What do you think is the role of community in times of crisis?**

2. The author grapples with his emerging identity as a "real runner" in this story. **How have your hobbies and interests shaped your identity and self-image?**

3. This story refers to many different numbers and metrics from the worlds of healthcare and running. **Are there significant numbers that relate to your life experiences?**

4. Technology plays an important role in the Hicks family's management of their pediatric cancer journey. **How have you used technology to manage life's ups and downs?**

5. A leukemia diagnosis catapulted the Hicks family into the world of pediatric cancer with perfect strangers. **Have you ever been thrown into a community of people with shared life experiences, good or bad?**

6. The author and his daughter each went through a personal transformation. **What has caused the most substantial transformations in your life? Your family's lives?**

7. The author refers to medical procedures and advances in the treatment of pediatric cancer. **Were you familiar with any of these advances before reading this book?**

8. The author decided to put pen to paper to capture his family's story. **Would you be willing to divulge your story to the world? Or would you keep your story a secret?**

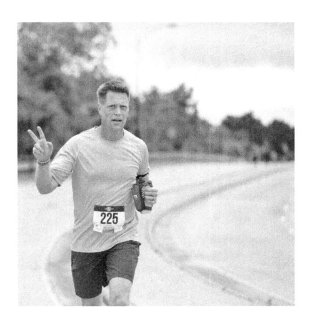

About the Author

Travis Lee Hicks is a father, husband, and long-distance runner who lives with his family of five in Greensboro, NC. A Middle Georgia native with a Master of Architecture from Princeton University, Hicks practiced architecture and design for 13 years before leaving the corporate world to teach interior architecture full-time at UNC Greensboro where he leads design students in community-engaged design projects that impact the greater Piedmont-Triad region.

Made in the USA
Middletown, DE
02 May 2021

38034764R00235